Drinking sea water

Using Dr. Hamer's 5 biological laws on self-healing

Drinking sea water

Using Dr. Hamer's 5 biological laws on self-healing

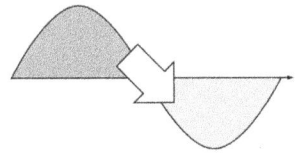

Francisco Martin

Why does the subtitle say "using Dr. Hamer's 5 biological laws on self-healing"?

When we are injured, symptoms like inflammation, tingling, redness, or heat appear. They don't make us worry because we know that they are healing symptoms of the injury.

Similarly, Dr. Hamer discovered that many illnesses are just the symptoms of recovery from previous overwork.

His discoveries allow us to make better use of sea water: to discover what we can expect from it in every situation.

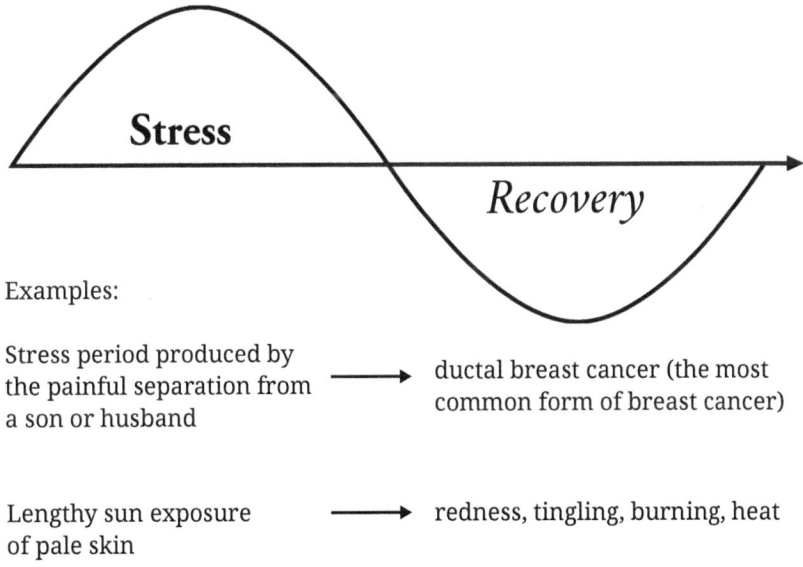

Examples:

Stress period produced by the painful separation from a son or husband ⟶ ductal breast cancer (the most common form of breast cancer)

Lengthy sun exposure of pale skin ⟶ redness, tingling, burning, heat

Acknowledgements

To Dr. Hamer for helping us
to better understand our bodies,

to René Quinton for discovering
the wonders of sea water,

to Dr. Maria Teresa Ilari who, in the land of Nicaragua,
fulfilled the dreams of Hamer and Quinton,

and to all those who have collaborated
in bringing sea water to everyone.

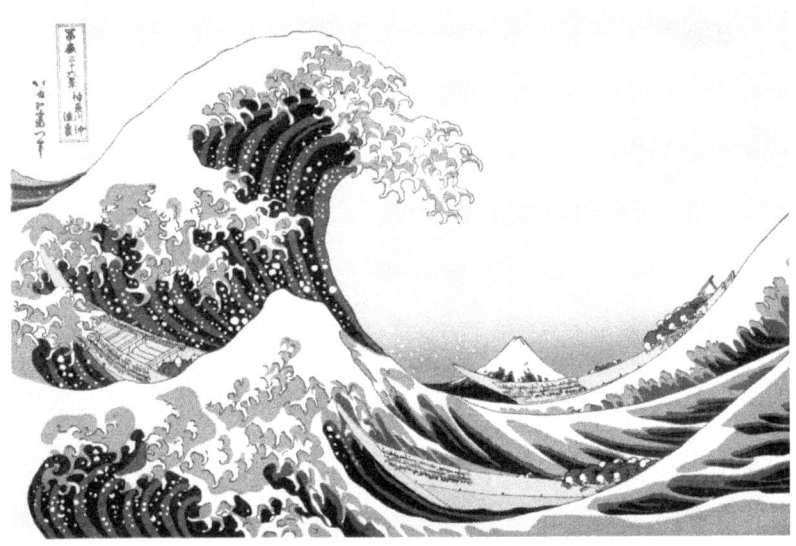

Sea water is a powerful remedy.
Drinking it according to Dr. Hamer's findings
   (that often when we have symptoms of illness we are already recovering)

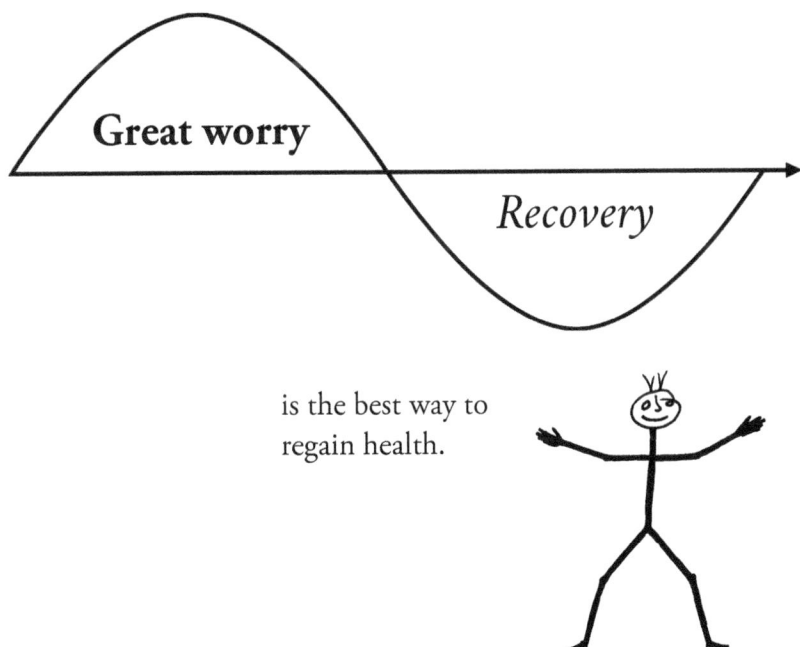

is the best way to regain health.

Chapter 1

History

How it all began

In ancient times, the Greeks and Romans praised the medicinal benefits of sea water.

In modern times, Richard Russell (1750) started to use sea water medicinally – for drinking and baths – in Brighton. His promising results attracted the Court; and thanks to that, Brighton became a city instead of being a fishermen's village.

At the beginning of 20th century, a lot of children in France were dying from cholera.

René Quinton saved them with injections of sea water.

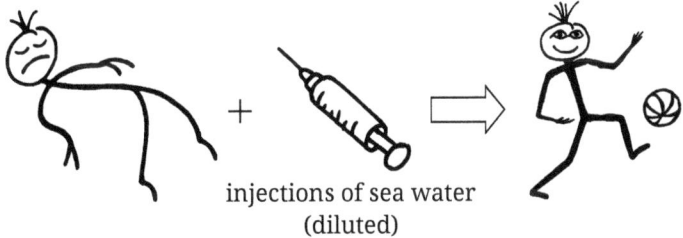

injections of sea water
(diluted)

From then on, and until 1980, it was prescribed by the French medical authorities (orally or injected).

From 1982, because of legal changes, it wasn't considered a medicine anymore. So, it cannot be injected legally intravenously in Europe (only as subcutaneous injections and under the personal responsibility of the doctor).

Why sea water is so effective as a cure

Because sea water (diluted) is identical to blood serum (without any organic component).

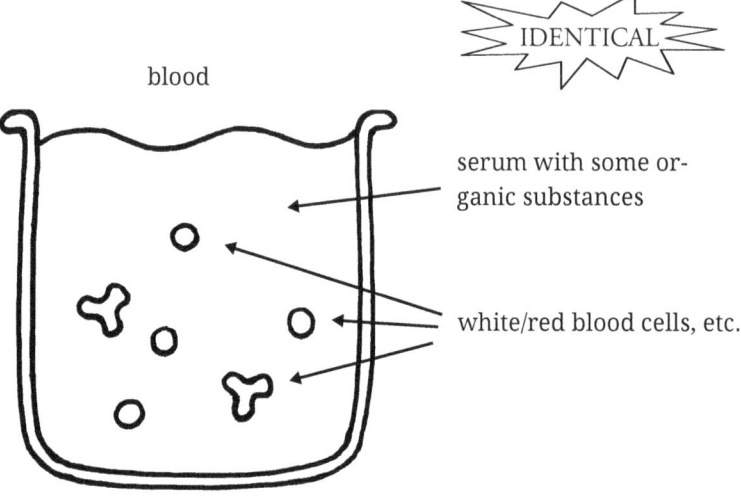

The Physicians' Desk Reference of 1975 in France (Dictionnaire Vidal) said:

> "René Quinton showed, in 1904, that Quinton® Isotonic is identical physically, chemically and physiologically to our inner medium, the one which provides the best conditions for life to isolated cells (in particular, red blood cells and white blood cells) and fragments of tissues."
>
> "It's possible to replace all the blood of an animal with Quinton® Isotonic without causing harm to it."

(Quinton® Isotonic is sea water diluted with spring water).

René Quinton's research

He discovered white blood cells can only live in sea water – once outside of the human body.

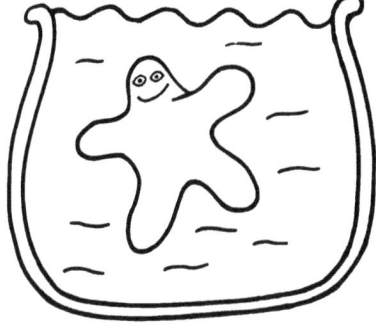
They live happily in sea water diluted with spring water.

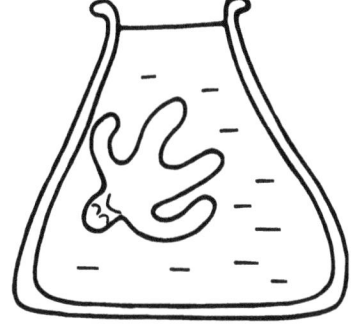
In any other place, they die.

Why did he try with white blood cells ?

Because they live isolated, far from other cells that could affect their behavior.

How to make isotonic sea water

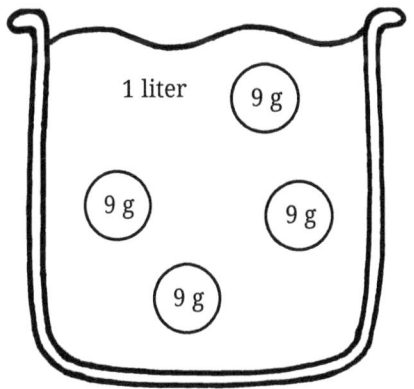

Sea water contains 36 grams of salt per liter.

(9 grams x 4 = 36 grams)

If we add 1 liter of sea water to 3 liters of spring water,

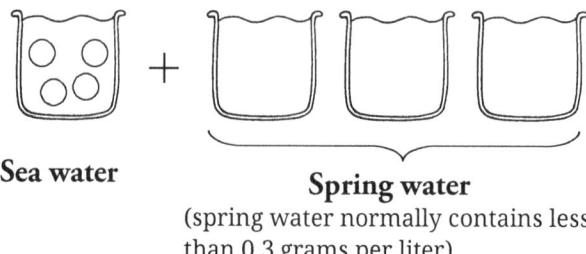

Sea water

Spring water
(spring water normally contains less than 0.3 grams per liter)

we obtain:

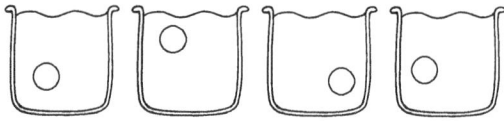

4 liters of **ISOTONIC sea water**, that means: with the same quantity of salts as blood (*9 g of salts per liter*).

> White blood cells live happily in this water and René Quinton injected it into the children who were dying from cholera.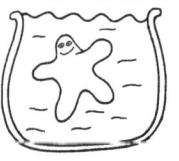

Quinton saved all the children with cholera but he didn't obtain such good results with other sickness, such as tuberculosis.

Thanks to Hamer we now understand why:

- Children with cholera were only intoxicated with contaminated food or water,

> and sea water cleans all poisonings.

- Hamer tells us tuberculosis is bacteria cleaning the body of cells that it built up during the former period of stress but now no longer needs.

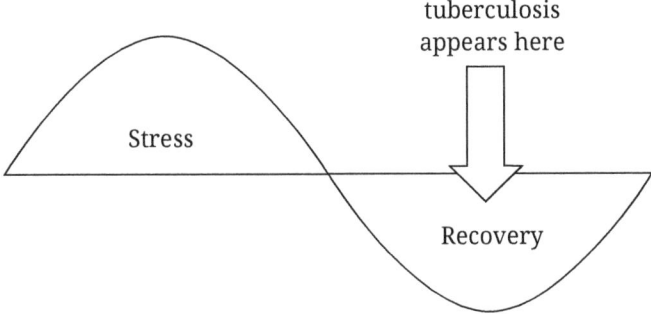

We must not eliminate bacteria.

> Tuberculosis bacteria are beneficial because they work as street-sweepers. Our bodies contain many beneficial bacteria – for example, in our intestines.

In these cases, we can drink sea water just to improve our well-being and accelerate the healing.

And if we don't want to suffer the symptoms again, we must avoid relapsing into a stress period.

> Not all stress periods gives rise to tuberculosis during recovery.

Tuberculosis is like the street-sweepers with their trucks taking everything that is no longer useful.

 **But then, why did people die from tuberculosis?**

Good question. We have to explain something more before we can give the answer.

17

Quinton tried to eliminate street-sweepers and garbage trucks.

Hamer explains why they came: we left paper or old stuff abandoned in the street.

And so, what do we have to do to avoid their reappearance with the noise of their trucks.

> When we are sick, we have to discover which worry made us ill, bear the healing symptoms the best we can and
> **try not to relapse into that worry.**

(Bear in the best way the annoyance of the current cleaning and no longer leave paper or old stuff in the street).

Summary

> Sea water will help us in any circumstance.

But, if we have just passed a big worry, it won't prevent our having all the symptoms that appear when the body is recovering.

We will feel them for fewer days, with better general feeling, but the body shows these symptoms when it is healing.

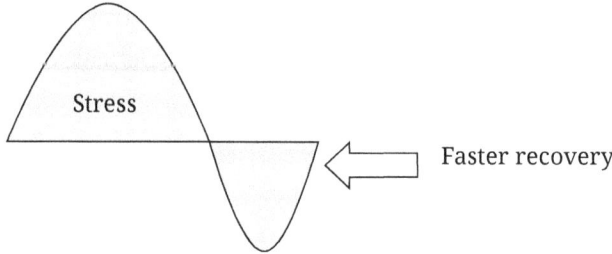

It's exactly the same as when works are being done to repair our road: we have to accept noise and annoyance for some days.

(If we don't allow them, we won't ever have the road in good condition.)

Chapter 2

Medical and nutritional use of sea water

We can use sea water:

- as food,
- as prevention,
- to detoxify,
- to resolve minor illnesses,
- as an aid in healing illnesses,
- for emergencies or terminally ill people.

As food

> The first instruction professional cycling teams give each new rider is: "You must drink sea water."

It's the best isotonic drink for athletes or when we sweat a lot.

- When we sweat, we lose salts that we can recover with sea water.

- In Nicaragua, people generally drink a quarter of a liter a day, because the temperature is high throughout the year.

We can use it as a substitute for salt in meals (see later its culinary use).

It also provides us with trace elements (gold, silver, copper), which are not present in refined salt.

> Processed foods (like bread), are usually made with refined salt (without trace elements). We can compensate for this micronutrient deficiency with sea water.

As prevention

By drinking sea water, we improve our general condition, and thus we will have a better state of mind to bear the inevitable setbacks of life (and not to get sick because of them).

It can also help us to avoid poisoning.

Examples:

- If we are well nourished with iodine by drinking sea water, our body won't need to assimilate more iodine, perhaps coming from a nuclear disaster. (This is why iodine tablets were distributed in Japan after Fukushima.)
- When we ask the dentist to remove mercury amalgams, it is recommended to drink sea water before and after the operation, and to rinse our mouths with it during the operation.[*]

In countries where there is a risk of child malnutrition, children are given three small glasses a day and this gives good results.

_____

(*) Swiss dentist who explains the use of sea water:
www.haroutunian.ch/depose_amalgames.htm

> In the chapter on Nicaragua we explain how, already in the early twentieth century, people drank it in distant coastal areas.

To detoxify

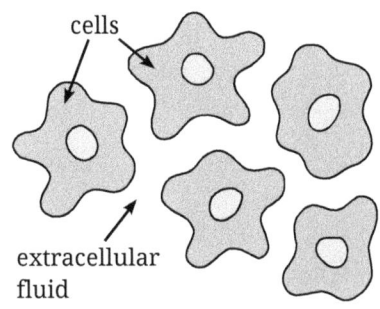

When we start to drink seawater, we feel an improvement in our general condition. We feel better and have more energy. All our body functions are restored.

This is because the cells of our body are bathed in a fluid and they work better when it is clean. Sea water is a supply of clean fluid that causes all cells to feel at their best.

> As with car engines, which give more power and use less fuel when we change the oil.

Sea water is particularly useful for cleaning this internal fluid when it's dirty, poisoned. Whether it is by:

- drinking or eating food with chemical additives,
- constantly having bad thoughts,
- living or working in contaminated environments,
- taking medication.

The latter is the case explained in the chapter devoted to veterinary use where a dying female dog, poisoned by drugs, heals in a few hours.

As an example of its cleansing power, the French medical handbook of 1975 said in the sea water's indications: "eliminates antibiotics".

The handbook also said it even washes out inherited defects: "Disappearance of physiological defects" (hereditary), and there are accounts of this use in the bibliography.[2]

We also intoxicate our bodies with internal secretions of adrenaline and other hormones when we have bad thoughts.

Trick

When we do things reluctantly, we have a feeling of discontent that harms our body and makes us very tired.

If we decide to do something, it is better to do it joyfully.

Externally, we can adopt the most appropriate attitude, but internally we can keep happy.

And so we will get less tired and we won't harm our body.

We poison ourselves by drugs, chemicals in drinks and food (like sugar or refined salt), bad thoughts or watching TV.

See more information on the book's website.

If we take sea water to detoxify us, then it's also important we avoid poisoning ourselves with all of the above.

To resolve minor illnesses

Minor complaints are easily resolved with sea water: gastritis, constipation, insomnia, cramps,... and also small wounds on the body or sores in the mouth heal better by washing them with sea water.

> Minor complaints can be indicators or the beginning of more serious diseases that we need to research.

As an aid in healing illnesses

The causes of our illnesses are:

- **Insufficient nutrition**: like the scurvy of sailors who didn't eat fruit and vegetables during their long trips.
- **Accidents**: trauma, burns, too intense efforts or exposing ourselves to environments when we are not used to them: sunburn on the beach or in high mountains, etc.
- **Poisoning**: usually due to medication.
- **Serious concerns**: which cause cancer, arthritis, cataracts, etc.

In the latter case, diseases have different symptoms when we are starting them (when we are still concerned), or when we have already resolved the concern and the body is recovering.

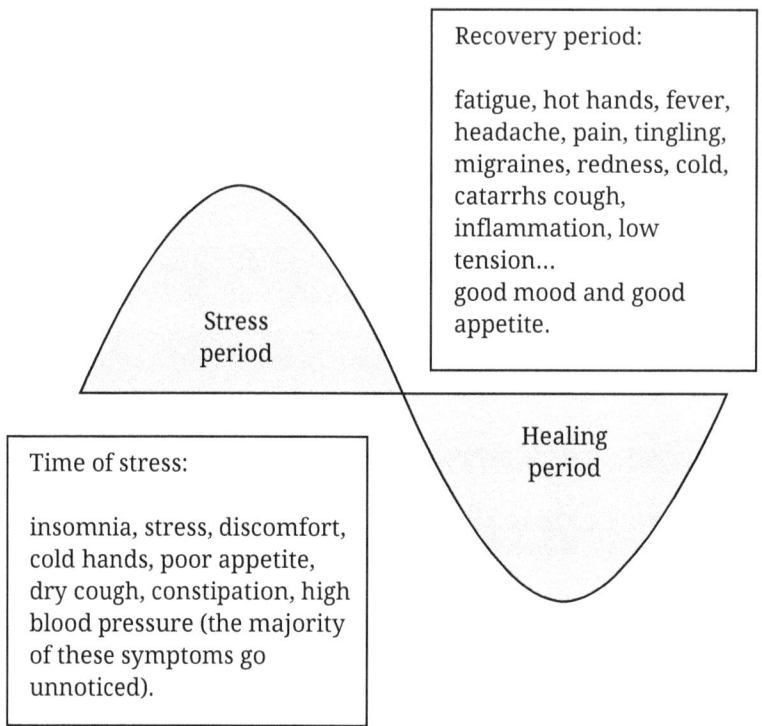

Often we don't pay attention to the discomfort of the first phase because we are obsessed with our concern. And so, we don't give importance to insomnia or lack of appetite.

> Who cares about eating or sleeping when we are pondering a serious problem all day long?

When we resolve the concern, the body begins to recover from the previous effort.

As we are no longer obsessed with our previous problem, we begin to pay attention to other things. We notice the symptoms the body is starting to produce and we mistakenly take them as the onset of an illness.

With Hamer's approach, we understand correctly what the body is doing and how it all started.

Hamer tells us by which emotional shock it all started and how each disease progresses. Therefore we know what to do, whether we are still in the preoccupying phase or whether we are already in the healing phase.

If we are still in the first phase, we must resolve the concern to begin healing.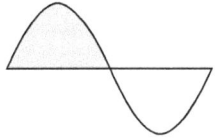

> Sea water, medicines and many other remedies can alleviate or eliminate the symptoms of the stress phase without solving the real cause.
> In these cases, we become a chronically ill person: we continually depend on a remedy or therapy.

> If we have a car tire that is losing air, we can inflate it every morning, or fix the puncture and forget about the problem.

If we are already in the healing phase, sea water will make it easier for us. In the most severe cases, large tumors, it may be necessary 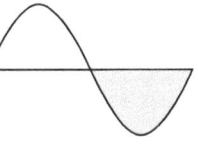 to take an anti-inflammatory medication. This is detailed further in the text.

For emergencies or terminally ill people

In the case of an emergency or terminally ill people, the use of (isotonic) sea water instead of the conventional physiologic saline solution, allows "miraculous" cures in a few hours, like those narrated by Quinton in the book *Le Plasma de Quinton*. In this book, we read how moribund children, dehydrated by cholera, or poisoned people recover their health in a few hours.

For transfusions, it has important advantages:

- There is no incompatibility of blood group.
- It's easier to get sea water than to find donors.
- It can be given to people who refuse transfusions.
- Avoids the risk of disease transmission.

How much should we take?

As a food, to prevent or resolve small diseases, we just need to take one or two tablespoons a day.

> If we take more, our bodies can begin important healing processes, which require an understanding of Hamer's approach so as not to confuse healing symptoms with an illness.

Once we have decided to drink plenty of sea water, there is no recommended dose, as we no longer take it as a medicine, but as a food or drink.

Do we count how much time we spend in the sun? No.

Only during the first days that we spend at the beach.

The same thing happens with sea water. Once we start taking it, and have passed our pending healing processes, we no longer measure how much we take.

In the same way that we don't count the potatoes or lettuces that we eat.

> As nutritional or preventive doses, Dr. Goizet recommended, in his 1871 book[6]:
> - Babies up to 6 months: a teaspoon (3 ml) mixed with milk.
> - Babies between 6 months and 1 year old: one teaspoon in the morning and in the afternoon.
> - One-year-old children: one teaspoon in the morning and two in the afternoon.
> - Children 2 to 3 years old: two teaspoons in the morning and in the afternoon.
> - Children from 4 to 7 years old: a small glass (50 ml) in the morning and in the afternoon.
> - Children from 8 to 11 years old: one small glass (50 ml) in the morning and two in the afternoon.
> - Young people from 12 to 15 years old: one medium glass (100 ml) in the morning and in the afternoon.
> - Adults: a large glass (150 ml) in the morning and in the afternoon.

The rule would be:

To take as much sea water as possible as long as the stool is soft but still shaped – it isn't liquid. Probably one or two glasses of sea water, without dilution, per day. We can take this diluted dose in drinks or in dishes during meals.

If we take too much, the feces become liquid, so we should stop drinking it or decrease the dose for a few days until they return to normal (and don't eat anything raw).

Summary

Sea water is ideal in some cases: dehydration, burns, poisoning, hemorrhages,... or in terminal situations.

Sea water is suitable for many people for its nutritious and detoxifying effects.

- Taken in small doses (one or two tablespoons of sea water per day) it is nutritious and cleansing without causing major healing processes (or showy symptoms: bone pain, headache, inflammation, tingling,...).

    Everything starts to work normally. We feel light and full of vitality.

- Higher doses require a calm decision from the patient, because perhaps he feels or senses, better than anyone, whether or not he should take it.

    Although many people who drink sea water do very well, it may not suit us (see the following paragraphs).

The more we take the more intense and short the cleansing or healing processes will be.

> (If we feel the healing symptoms, such as headaches, and want to alleviate them, we should take less seawater and refresh our head. See the detail of this information in Chapter 9: "Therapeutic guide for the patient".)

The use of sea water is risky in the following cases:

- When the patient doesn't know Hamer's approach and can confuse the healing symptoms with a new illness.
- Those described by Hamer as being difficult to treat: such as certain serious or complex psychological problems.
- When the person has suffered from a prolonged or intense concern and the effort required to heal is greater than that which the body can provide (see Chapter 9).

> In these cases, healing should be slowed down so that the patient's energy doesn't run out.

For added security, we should go see a doctor who knows Hamer's approach.

Experts can help find out how intense and long the healing phase will be, and whether it is appropriate to take medication to slow down the process.

Warning:

When we don't have a clear disease (like cancer), but our body is not working well, the origin is usually in the teeth, and we will recover just (and only) by fixing them. It is very important to read about this topic on the book's website.

Chapter 3

Practical aspects

How to take it?

We can bathe or introduce it into the body through any opening without any problem.

> The only thing we shouldn't do is **wash the inside of the nose daily with sea water without diluting.**
>
> Occasionally we can use it without diluting, but not daily.

We can drink it, rinse our mouths, put it on our eyes, wash our ears, etc.

> If we heat sea water above 111 °F, it loses its best properties.
> If we only want it to be less cold, we must heat it to the 'bain-Marie'(*), stirring continuously, and stopping it before, by putting our finger inside, it burns us.
> Things burn us when they are above 111 °F.

(*) We can also heat the water in an incubator (see Appendix C: "Homemade inventions").

Orally

We can drink it as it is in the sea or diluted.

Remember that if we mix a glass of sea water with three glasses of fresh water, we obtain isotonic sea water, which has the same amount of salt as the fluids in our body.

Since it has the same amount of salts as our body, we neither find it salty nor bland nor make us thirsty.

When we have salty drinks or foods we get thirsty. The body asks us to compensate for that excess salt with fresh water or fruit or vegetables.

> (This is explained in detail at the end of Appendix A: "Scientific basis".)

> Sick, aged people or babies drinking sea water may not realize that their bodies are asking for fresh water.
> In this case, it is better to give them isotonic water.

Instead, we can drink as much isotonic sea water as we like and it won't make us thirsty.

> **How to prepare the best sport (isotonic) drink**
>
> - We mix in a bottle, three quarters of a liter of fresh water with a quarter of a liter of sea water.
> - We may add a little natural juice or panela to give it more flavor.

It's the best isotonic drink because it's the closest thing to the fluid that bathes the cells of our body. In this isotonic drink, the cells of our body live in the best way – as Quinton verified with white blood cells. In any other medium, they die.

Whichever way we drink it, it's best to keep it in our mouth several seconds before swallowing it.

The ideal is to dilute it with saliva and swallow it when we no longer notice it's salty.

> Something from the food is absorbed in the mouth. In India they call it "prana", and that is why everyone recommends chewing and not swallowing food until we have absorbed all its flavor. If we are eating an exquisite delicacy, why swallow it before it stops giving us flavor?
>
> We can also verify that we absorb something through the mouth when we drink an alcoholic drink, the effects of which we feel shortly after drinking it, a long time before it is assimilated by the intestine.
>
> Or when dentists must take special caution when removing amalgams so that the patient doesn't absorb mercury through the palate.
>
> Likewise, homeopathic medicines are absorbed through the mouth.

Sea water is diuretic. We shouldn't take it before a bus trip or going to a concert.

And the more we take (either diluted or as it is), the softer is the stool.

We can also add a very small amount to the water we normally drink.

If we drink bottled water, we can add a small amount to the bottle, this way we don't have to add it every time we drink from it.

This small amount even improves the taste of water and is provides trace elements that fresh water would not otherwise have, especially if we drink distilled or reverse osmosis water.

When drinking tap water, we can fill bottles and add sea water to them.

Sea water reduces the appetite (if we take it before meals).

But we don't know anyone who lives only drinking sea water.

> It seems that, in this sense, people are capable of incredible things, such as those who live without eating or drinking anything or just by drinking.
>
> In Europe, famous are the cases of Therese Neumann or Saint Nicholas of Flüe, who lived only by receiving the sacrament of communion daily. But as it appears in P. Straubinger's documentary (www.light-documentary.com), this happens in various cultures of the world and also among people who are not especially religious.

It is possible to subsist only with sea water for a time in exceptional cases (shipwrecks, catastrophes,...).

Researchers have demonstrated the benefits for castaways of drinking sea water in **small sips** to survive longer at sea.

Rinses and dental washing

We can use it to brush our teeth and rinse our mouths.

Also to heal mouth sores.

In the case of teeth with advanced cavities (with which we have already sensitivity), rinsing with sea water serves as a **temporary** remedy.

And in these cases, every time we take acid food or acid liquids (with a pH less than 7, like lemon, wine or beer), we have to rinse our mouths with sea water.

The state of the teeth is the first thing we have to look at when we have a health problem (except for cancers, the origin of which is always the one indicated by Hamer).

As long as we have cavities, teeth in poor condition and especially those with root canal treatment causing our illness, any treatment will be unsuccessful.

> **Warning**
>
> Let's recall what Dr. Ernest Adler said about the harm of devitalized teeth (perform "root canal treatment", "endodontics").
>
> (And Weston A. Price said it already a century ago – www.westonaprice.org)
>
> Let's not try to eliminate with sea water the symptoms (a fistula, a pain) indicating a hidden problem, that we don't see: a devitalized tooth which affects the functioning of the organs which share its same meridian (see the book's website and [4]).

By injection

(Let's remember that it is not legal to inject it intravenously in the European Union.)

The most common form of applying it is subcutaneous injection.

In general, René Quinton recommended a minimum dose of 700 ml of isotonic sea water every five days for an adult. (Between one hundredth and one hundredth and a half of body weight.)

For specific applications, doses are mentioned in his books and on the Canadian website cited at the end of this chapter.

The details of the procedure are explained in Appendix B:

"How to give subcutaneous injections".

In severe cases or for emergencies (hemorrhages), liters of isotonic sea water (because it is identical to blood serum) can be injected without affecting the kidneys. In these cases, sea water is injected intravenously (see Chapter 5: "Frequently asked questions", dealing with this subject).

Through the anus

To absorb it, not to wash the intestines

We can use a 50 ml syringe to which we connect the cannula of a pear enema. (The syringe and the pear are sold in pharmacies, the plastic tube in a hardware store.)

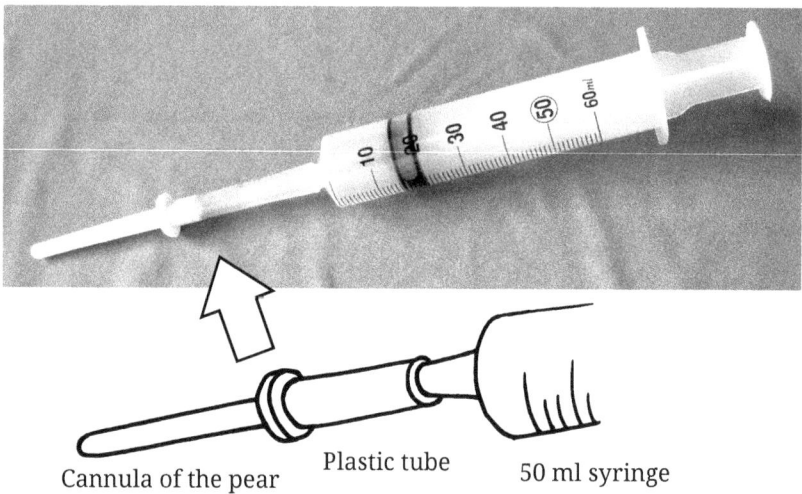

Cannula of the pear   Plastic tube   50 ml syringe

With the syringe we can control very well the quantity that we introduce. If we introduce too much undiluted sea water, the body expels it in no time.

In the case of undiluted water, it is advisable to introduce very little (5 ml).

In the case of isotonic sea water we can introduce large quantities (250 ml) and it is easy to resist its expulsion. In this case we can simply use a pear enema.

Advantages of this method: it's as effective and has an effect almost as fast as an IV injection, because water must not pass through the digestive tract. This method is easy and quick to perform and allows the introduction of large quantities of isotonic sea water.

Wash our intestines (colon cleansing)

Even though we can use isotonic sea water to do a "colon enema", the method called Shank Prakshalana (from India) is much more effective because it washes all the intestines, not just the colon.

It consists of drinking small glasses of isotonic sea water at body temperature, while we make simple movements to ease its progress through the digestive tract.

And so on, until the water coming out of the anus is as clean as the one we drink (approximately after drinking 4 liters in 4 to 5 hours).

Since this method doesn't require special devices, it has the advantage (compared to colon enema) that it can be performed at home.

(More information on the book's website.)

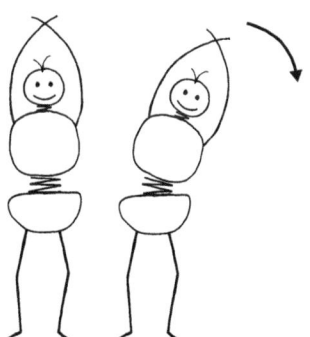

Into the eyes

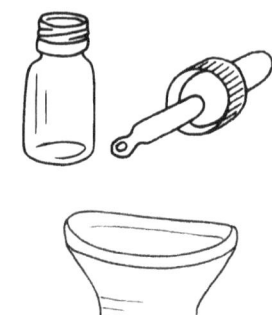

We can put drops in our eyes with an eye dropper, use an eye bath or we can use swimming goggles contrariwise. Instead of using them in the pool to keep water out of our eyes, we use them out of the water so that the water we put in doesn't come out.

We fill them with sea water and adjust them well to the eyes, with the elastic bands tight so that the water doesn't come out. We can use isotonic or undiluted sea water. The best seems to be to use it without dilution, like when we open our eyes swimming in the sea.

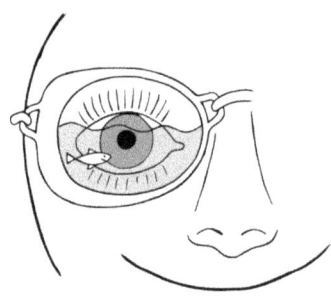

The eyes are another privileged entry door to the body (like the mouth and anus). That's why we can take medicines through them. Specially for eye ailments, but also for body ones when the rest of the entry points are unusable (for example, with unconscious patients).

Sprayed

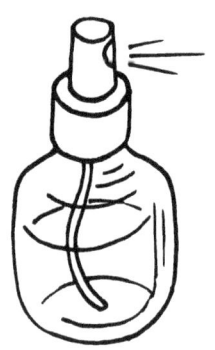

We can use a small sprayer in any location.

If we spray sea water in a room, we will absorb it through the nose. If we spray it on the skin, it refreshes us.

Coastal residents breathe it continuously in this way as the sea breeze carries droplets of sea water. This is why iron oxidizes so much on the coast. The same goes for sea voyages.

Washing the inside of the nose

Traditionally in India, they do what they call "Jala Neti", that consist of using a teapot to introduce water into one nostril and expel it through the other, but it is more practical to use a syringe like the one described above.

For occasional use we can dilute it by half.

> For daily use we must use isotonic sea water.

> Doctor Pros's clinic in Barcelona offers various treatments with sea water spray for respiratory and ear diseases – www.doctorpros.com.

Ear irrigation

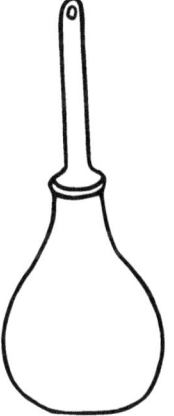

To wash the earwax plugs from the ear canals, while standing, we introduce the sea water with a small pear enema or syringe without a needle and let it come out normally. We apply it three times a day and the sea water will dissolve the earwax.

We can also put a few drops in the ear canal before bed, so that the wax dissolves; and lie down on the side opposite the blocked duct.

Bath

When we bathe in the sea, we absorb water through the skin in the same way that we absorb any cream we apply to ourselves.

If we use oils and creams that don't go away with water, we prevent our skin from absorbing sea water.

If we want to take warm sea water baths at home, we can build an "ofuro" (see Appendix C).

Hair loss

Doctor Goizet's book describes the case of a person who had completely lost his hair. During a five-month voyage at sea, he showered twice a day with sea water, and he rubbed his head, in the morning and in the afternoon, with sea water. At the end of the trip, his head was covered with abundant hair.

(See the full mention on the book's website.)

How to get it

We can take it from any beach where it looks clean and doesn't smell bad.

If we take it during the bathing season there may be sunscreens floating on the surface of the water. To avoid them, we immerse a bottle closed and, under water, we open it and let it fill.

If we can stock up before the bathing season, we spare ourselves this care.

Near the mouth of rivers and big cities, it is better not to take it.

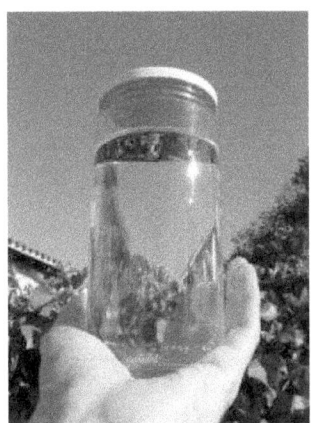

Example of sea water, transparent and clean, taken from the beach. Without any filtration or treatment.

If we have a boat or someone can bring it to us from out to sea, that's better.

But anyway, the water from the beach has all the properties.

Conservation

It keeps indefinitely out of the sun and without a cooler.

It will spoil and smell if, when we take it, it contains a lot of algae and we don't filter it. If it's in this state, we can give it to the plants by diluting it with tap water.

Where to buy it

Here is provided only general information. The most up-to-date information is available on the book's website.

Sea water ampoules are sold in pharmacies in many countries (at $ 30 US a quarter of a liter). These ampoules have a pharmacological quality bottling process.

In several countries there are companies that bottle and sell much cheaper sea water. They all sell it filtered. Some of them treat sea water in several other ways: ozonization, ion exchange (to reduce the amount of Boron), or even desalination. It is better to drink sea water with the least possible treatment. The price of sea water from these bottling companies is about $2 US a liter.

In France

- techsealab.com (shop: oceanik.fr)
- source-claire.com (Quinton® products)
- laboratoires-superdiet.fr (search "Oligocean")
- csbs-odemer.fr

In Canada

- oceanplasma.net (warning: ozonized, not recommended by the EFSA. More information on the book's website)
- shopbiocean.com (Biocean®, $82 US / liter)

In Italy

- aquamarina.info
- marentia.it
- steralmar.it (warning: ion exchange processed)

In Spain

- aguademar.com.es (the first and the biggest company)
- aquademar.eu
- aguademarsietemares.com (warning: ion exchange processed)
- quinton.es (pharmaceutical quality bottling) $100US / liter
- aguademar.es (warning: ion exchange processed)
- augasdemar.com
- ibizayformenteraaguademar.com
- rioka.es

In Germany

- biomaris.com $10 US / liter

In Mexico

- facebook.com/AguaDeMarEmbotellada
- quintonmexico.com

In Colombia

- amarisagua.com

In Argentina

- pranamaraguademar.com

In U.S.A.

- quicksilverscientific.com

In different countries (U.S.A., Japan, Brazil) partially desalinated sea water is sold.

It can be useful to people living far from the sea, or who don't yet know the benefits of natural sea water.

Their websites are:

- destinydeepseawater.com (U.S.A.)
- 63water.com (Brazil)
- ako-kasei.co.jp (Japan)

Information in internet

- **oceanplasma.org**
  Doctors in Canada using sea water.

- **the-savoisien.com/wawa-conspi/ viewtopic.php?id=1937**
  Website containing addresses of doctors who use sea water in France to treat herniated discs.

- **youtube.com**
  Dr. Epineuze's videos showing the application of subcutaneous injections to cure non-operated herniated discs (search *Epineuze*).

- **drinkingseawater.com** (companion website).

Chapter 4

Cooking with sea water

Traditionally, many countries use sea water in their cooking.

- The French Bouillabaisse.
- The paella of Valencia (Spain).
- Norman fishermen and their mackerel cooked in sea water.(*)
- The fishermen of Southern Italy and their *freselle* or *frisa* (unsalted buns baked twice), that they wet with sea water before eating.
- Boiled octopus ("pulpo á feira") in Galicia (Spain).
- Wrinkled potatoes ("papas arrugás") in the Canary Islands.

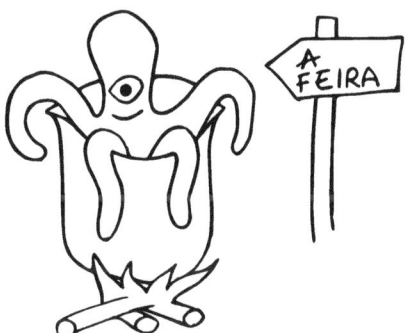

Currently it'is used in many restaurants to cook fish or seafood (or to wash them).

The flavor of dishes prepared with sea water is better than those prepared with sea salt.

(*) chezmonpoissonnier.fr/recette-traditionnelle-bouonia-maquereaux/

When we don't live near the coast, it is more expensive to cook daily with it, especially if we boil it (and part of it evaporates).

In a later section, some 'tricks' are explained for cooking without boiling the sea water. That way we obtain two benefits:

- If we don't heat it above body temperature (which will scald us), it maintains its best properties.
- Nothing is lost through evaporation so less sea water needed.

To cook with it we must take into account the quantity of water in the ingredients (and not to add salt, of course).

That is to say:

- If we make a stew of potatoes and marrow (mature zucchini), we use half of sea water and half fresh water, because the potatoes and the marrow are ingredients that contain a lot of water.

    Once we have lightly fried all the ingredients (garlic, onion, potato, etc.), we add fresh water and sea water so that it covers everything. We cook the marrow and other soft vegetables for less time than the other tougher ingredients, adding them just before the cooking of the other ingredients is complete.
- To make paella using only rice (which contains no water), we use one part sea water to five parts fresh water. To make a vegetable paella, we use sea water and fresh water half-and-half because the vegetables contain water.
- Beans should be cooked without salt and then when ready, seasoned with sea water.

Drinks and cold dishes

Citric fruit juices

- The acid of citric fruit (lemon, orange, grapefruit), masks the bitterness of sea water.

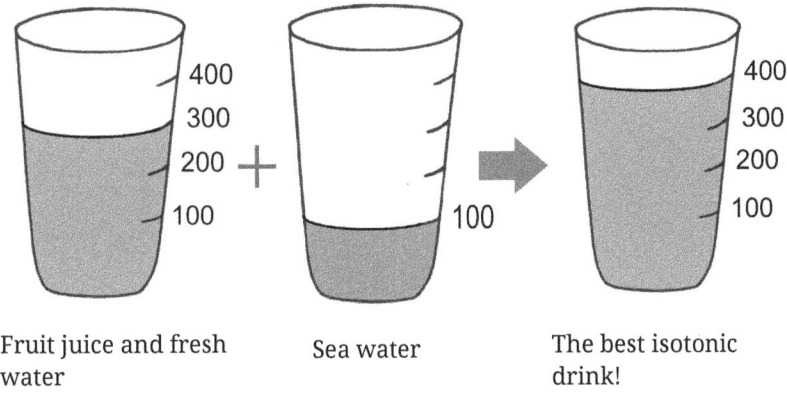

Fruit juice and fresh water   Sea water   The best isotonic drink!

The best proportions are three to one - 300 ml fruit juice + fresh water; 100 ml sea water. Any greater concentration of sea water will simply make us thirsty.

This way, we are preparing the best isotonic drink we can ever imagine.

If we want to sweeten it, we don't add sugar. We may add jaggery ("panela", "rapadura", "piloncillo") which is the unrefined juice of sugar cane, a much more healthy sweetener than refined sugar since it contains natural vitamins and minerals. It is sold in 'fair trade' shops (more information in book's web).

Sangria

- It is made as any other citric fruit juice. Just add red wine.

Beer

- If we add a very small quantity (drops) of sea water to beer, it improves its taste. If this improved taste leads us to over indulge we can ease the hangover next day by drinking sea water. (It shouldn't be an excuse to drink too much.)

Gazpacho

A traditional Andalusian soup served cold. Make in the summer when the ingredients are at their best. Serves four to six.

Ingredients: 1/4 cucumber, 1 red pepper, 225g/8oz tomatoes, 1 small onion, 1 garlic clove, a few sprigs of parsley, pepper to taste.

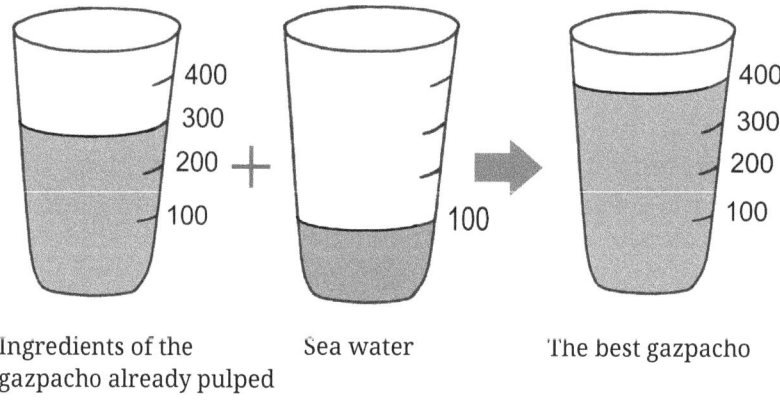

Ingredients of the gazpacho already pulped   Sea water   The best gazpacho

- Chop roughly all the ingredients and blend them in a liquidizer goblet. Add the third part of sea water, chill and serve with croûtons.

Sandwiches

- Use unsalted bread (bread is usually made with refined salt) and add sea water.

Salads

- We can season them with sea water instead of salt.

In sandwiches and salads, it's best to use a sprayer to control the quantity we use; and it's better to apply the sea water before other dressings since oil and sauces prevent sea water from impregnating the food effectively.

Hot dishes

> Since sea water loses its best properties when heated above 111 °F (44 °C), we should employ the following "**trick**":
>
>> The food should be cooked with the sauce very concentrated; once cooked and cooled below 111 °F add sea water to the desired consistency.

Some thermometers measure the heat that things emit without touching them (see Appendix C for more details).

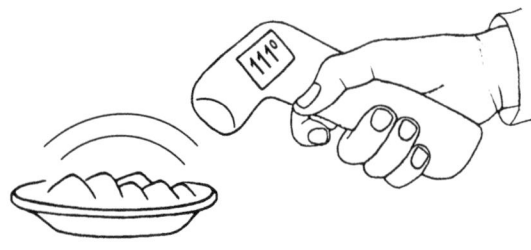

If we use them, we need to thoroughly stir the food before measuring. Otherwise, we will measure only the surface temperature and inside can be much hotter.

> We shouldn't use medical thermometers since they are not designed to operate above 111 °F and are easily broken.

Puree of potatoes

- Prepare steamed potatoes (or if boiled, drain thoroughly).
- Mash them while they cool down.
- When cooled to 111 °F, add sea water. A good consistency is creamy: neither liquid nor very dense.
- We may dress the potatoes with a bit of olive oil and parsley as a garnish.

Porridge (oatmeal or cornmeal mush)

- We boil the cereal with little water.
- When we move it away from the fire, we wait until it cools down and then we add sea water.

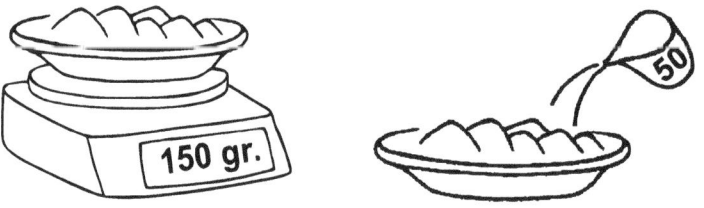

If we have 150 grams of porridge, we add 50 grams of sea water. It is a delicious porridge.

Garlic soup

- We make garlic soup by frying the garlic as usual, and then adding fresh water and breadcrumbs to the fried garlic (better unsalted breadcrumbs, of course). It is best to make a very thick mixture and then,
- when it has cooled down sufficiently (111 °F), we add sea water.

Fried banana

- Slice and fry banana to the preferred consistency. Allow to cool, then add sea water and stir well. The sweetness of banana masks the bitterness of sea water.

Soup

- We can prepare any soup using unsalted stock, and, once cooled add to it a third part of sea water.

> The general rule is that we can add a third part of sea water to the food that we have prepared (and don't add salt, of course).

Other practicalities in the kitchen

Use sea water, rather than salinated water:

- To prepare table olives.
- To steep dried chickpeas before cooking.

Try also having a bottle of sea water at the dinner table so that those dining can season their food to taste.

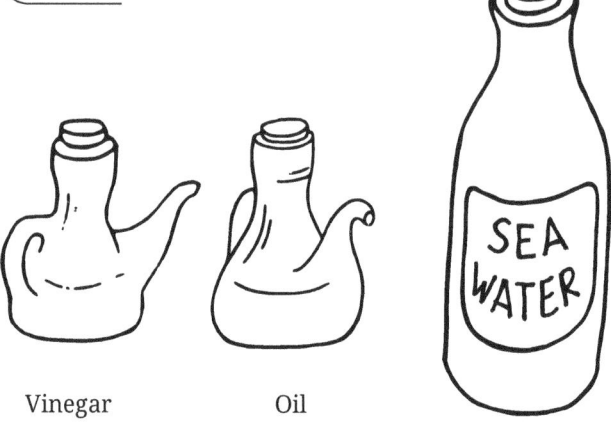

Vinegar   Oil

Chapter 5

Frequently asked questions

I feel good. If I take sea water, will I notice anything?
The better you feel, the fewer effects you will notice.

If we mix sea water with juices or dilute it, does it lose its effectiveness?

No. It only loses its powerful properties if we heat it above 111°F (40 °C). (That is the maximum temperature we can take it without being scalded.)

Is so much salt good for kidneys or for blood pressure?
Tests performed on geriatric patients, where many have high blood pressure, show that it normalizes blood pressure and is a diuretic. Medical texts also state that kidneys need sodium (as found in sea water) to function.

In experiments with dogs, which were injected with large quantities of diluted sea water, researchers found that kidneys were able to eliminate sixty times more urine than was normal; and that there were no harmful long-term effects on the health of the animal (see Appendix A: "Scientific basis").

Does the medical use of sea water have any harmful side effects?
The French physicians' desk reference book of 1975 [3] says that it doesn't have contraindications.

However, if we take daily more than a couple of spoonfuls, then we can trigger an important process of cure, which has its own symptoms, and we must know the approach of Dr. Hamer in order to understand this process completely.

But the doctor has recommended me not to take so much salt
We must make sure that the doctor knows the difference between refined salt and marine salt – the one used by our ancestors.

In Japan[*], cases of hypertension increased after they banned by law the production of sea salt.

Does water lose its properties by transporting it?
It's a sensible question. For example, wine producers know that wine doesn't taste the same at sea level as it does at altitude, and that it's important to let it settle after transportation.

Historical medical experiments show that sea water has the same properties before and after transport.

But the water of the sea is polluted
There are two types of contamination:

- Biological contamination caused by microbes.
- Contamination caused by chemical products.

The biological contamination of sea water only occurs near river mouths, because salt kills any microbe in a short time. Any biologist knows that it is impossible to cultivate pathogens in sea water.

For instance, in the Dead Sea, because it is so saline, it kills very rapidly any living microbes that enter from the river Jordan.

(*) http://web.ako-kasei.co.jp/en/column/umigaanatawokaeru/index.html
In the event of this website having changed, the information can be found by searching for "1971 site:ako-kasei.co.jp" with your web search engine.

> There is something special about the sea, and it is that, although the sea is full of bacteria, none of them are harmful to man or animal. Sea only kills bacteria that are harmful to animals or man. It is incredible, but it is true.

Concerning the contamination by chemical products, the sea gets rid of them at the surface and at depth.

- At the surface, those which are less dense evaporate, or are destroyed by sun light.
- At depth, heavier elements sink out of danger because of their density.
    In the same way that sediments rapidly sink to the bottom of the bucket if we collect sea water on the beach.

What will happen to me if I drink too much (half a liter of pure sea water), suddenly?
First, it will make you thirsty (for fresh water).

Obviously, drink what your body demands: 3 times the amount of undiluted sea water ingested.

Probably it will give you diarrhea. Stop drinking sea water, and in one day or two, the diarrhea will clear up. It is not recommended to drink too much sea water because it unnecessarily irritates the intestines.

If we want to clean them, we had better use isotonic water.

What will happen to me if I drink a lot (one liter) of diluted sea water (isotonic)?
The worse you are feeling, the more improvement you will notice in your overall wellbeing.

What will happen to me if I inject myself with too much (liters)?
Idem: the worse you are feeling, the more improvement you will notice in your overall wellbeing.

You can inject yourself with several liters of isotonic sea water without harmful effects.

> If you feel good and inject yourself with 250 ml, you won't feel anything.
>
> It's like cleaning a window that's already clean. Will we see any change? No.
>
> Obviously, if you inject it subcutaneously in a short time, it will form a bump the size of a tennis ball that will take a few hours to disappear.

The animals which have been injected with sea water (without dilution), in great quantity (200 ml to a dog of 10 Kg), are immobilized for some time. The more that is injected, the more time they lay. Then they drink triple the quantity that has been injected. When they get up, they are rejuvenated.

In Appendix A, titled "Scientific basis", we can read about the experiments that René Quinton made with dogs. In them, he used isotonic sea water.

Is it best to inject sea water intravenously, subcutaneously or take orally?

The effect is the same irrespective of the way that we take it.

It is just a question of convenience and of how quickly we want to feel the effects.

I have a herniated disc, sciatica, back pain... Can sea water help me?

Doctor François Epineuze cured 100% of these diseases simply by injecting 250 ml of isotonic sea water subcutaneously, around the affected vertebrae, in one, two or three sessions. The result wasn't as good when they have previously undergo surgery (see his videos on www.youtube.com). Doctors who perform these injections call it "percutaneous hydrotomy".

If we dissolve marine salt[(*)] *or rock salt in water, does this have the same effect as sea water?*

We've always used the medicinal properties of inland saline water, like the water of Carabaña in Spain or that of the Great Salt Lake in the U.S.A.

Sea salt (and sea water) is used in many medicines, whether modern or traditional (Ayurvedic).

For example, the most widely used homeopathic remedy, Natrum Muriaticum, is sea salt. (Currently most manufacturers of this remedy use refined salt instead of sea salt. Only one uses sea salt just like Hahnemann – the inventor of homeopathy – did).

If we don't have sea water, water with sea salt or rock salt is a good substitute[(**)], but it doesn't have all the properties of sea water. For example, white blood cells can only live in diluted (isotonic) sea water, while in any other artificial sea water, they die.

I am Muslim. Is sea water Halal?
The Islamic Cultural Centre of Valencia (Spain) certifies that the sea water contained in the products Quinton® is Halal (authorized for the consumption for Muslims).

Is it possible that sea water hurts me? It seems to me that I get a headache when I drink it, or pain in my bones, or...
We may think that sea water 'hurts us' when we drink it because we don't know Dr. Hamer's discoveries, because we are confusing the cure symptoms with an illness, (headaches, inflammations, itching, are typical symptoms of the recovery phase, according to Dr. Hamer's discoveries). We should consult a doctor or therapist who knows Dr. Hamer's approach. Later there is a chapter explaining the case of a person for whom sea water was (initially and apparently) harmful.

(*) Unfortunately, marine salt is very similar to refined salt (see book's website).
(**) "The sodium chloride treatment, without being the true marine treatment, therefore already approaches it singularly." [1c]

> Not all the pains appear during the recovery phase. There are illnesses in which pain appears in the stress phase, such as in the case of ulcers, angina pectoris, etc.

Are the proprietary brands of sea water sold in pharmacies, or brands that have been bottled in special locations any better than what we can pick up at the beach?
Experience indicates that sea water from any source is equally good.

Does the water of all the seas and oceans have the same effect?
Concerning their medicinal effects, it seems so. The taste is another question.

You can drink the water of the Atlantic or Pacific very easily. This is not the case of Mediterranean water. It is more difficult to swallow without dilution because it is more salty than that with the oceans.

However, that is not sufficient reason for people who live beside the Mediterranean, to buy it from the Atlantic.

It seems that nature provides us what we need at each time and place:

- Fruit comes in the summer, when we sweat more and we need to restore more liquid.
- The figs of a dry place have less water than those of the coast. Maybe it is this way because in a dry place, we sweat less and we need less water in the fruit.

For that reason, the food that grows near us is probably best for us.

Which water should we use to dilute sea water?
You may use the same one that you use for drinking.

How long does it take to feel the effect of taking sea water?
The effect is immediate. Generally, in a few hours the whole body's wellbeing is increased.

I take medication; will sea water suit me?
Sea water will help you to overcome the side effects of the medication and it will serve you as a general regenerator.

Here we recommend drinking sea water with an understanding of the approach of Dr. Hamer, who only used other medications in a very few percentage of cases.

Is there any case in which sea water doesn't produce any effect?
Yes, when the one that takes it is in a good health condition, or when the sick person takes too little [2].

I am vegetarian. May I take sea water?
The sea water (not micro filtered) contains a multitude of living organisms (algae, bacteria), but these are not animals, and therefore, you can eat them.

Does sea water have the same effect for animals as it does for people?
Yes.

Chapter 6

Medical approach of Dr. Hamer

(An introduction)

If I go to a party wearing some very beautiful but uncomfortable shoes

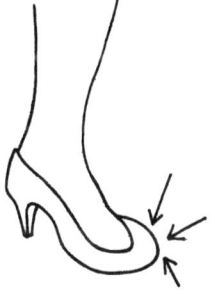

I'll end up with this area of the foot: red, with pain, heat, and a bit inflamed.

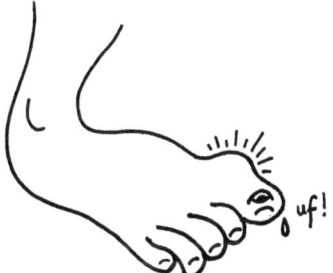

Are we sick? No.
Our foot is sick? No.

We say **no** because we know what has happened.

> Our DESIRE to wear these shoes to the party is the cause of the wound.

When the same happens us at any other place on the skin, we say 'we are sick'.

> The only difference is: in the first case we knew the reason, and we don't in the second.

When the same happens inside our body, we also say 'we are sick'. Because we don't know the cause.

> Hamer tells us, for each sickness, what was the originating thought.

And besides that, any expert can see, just looking at the CT (radiography) of our brain.

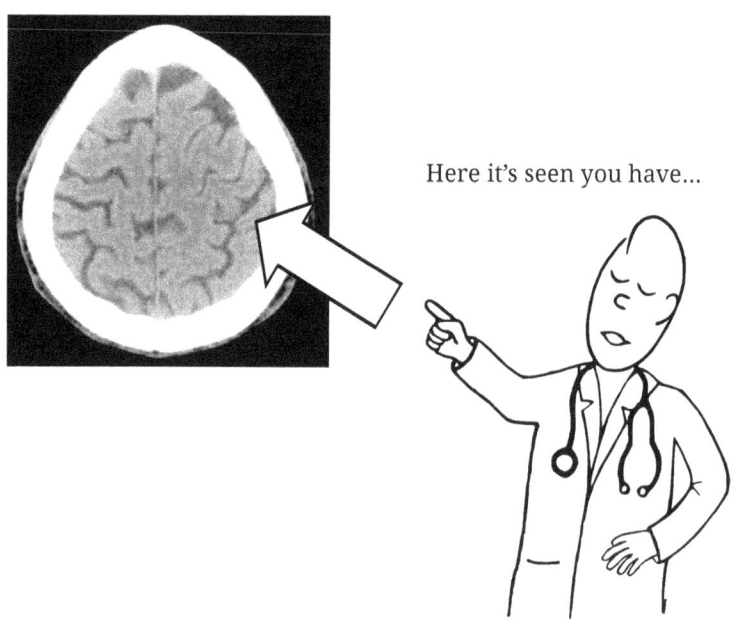

Here it's seen you have...

when we have these symptoms:

- pain
- heat
- redness
- inflammation

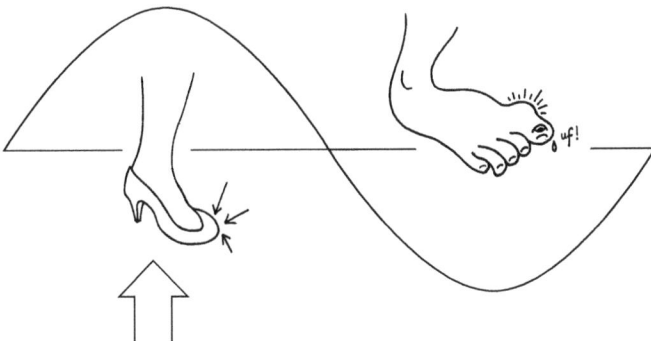

it's because **before** we have being **forcing** the body by a desire.

The same happens with diseases:

Ductal breast cancers, (the most common form of breast cancer), are **inflammations** that appear at this time.

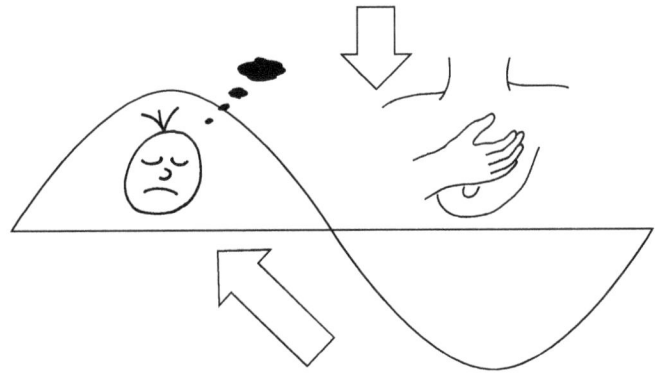

They appear because **before** we have being forcing the body by feeling overwhelmed by the separation from a loved one.

What to do, in these cases?

> Leave the body to finish its healing phase and avoid relapsing into the worry.
> (Do not wear those shoes for some time.)

We don't feel internal wounds as much as skin ones because the skin has many more nerve endings.

But inner wounds are exactly as the ones produced by a tight shoe.

> Thoughts are the cause of many diseases.

the more serious the concern is and the more it lasts, the longer and more visible the recovery will be.

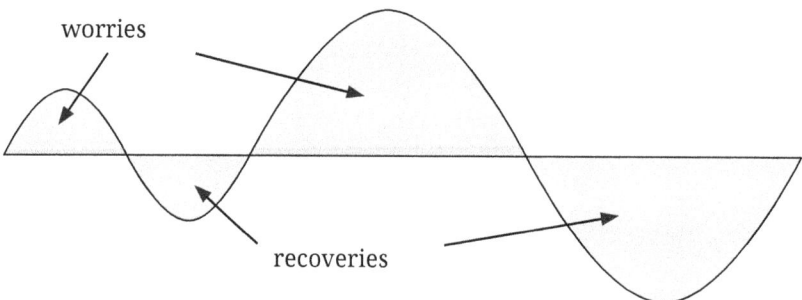

This is why it is worth resolving problems as soon as possible.

> **The approach of Hamer...**
>
> ... helps us for all the more common serious illnesses:
> - cancer
> - heart problems
> - osteoporosis
> - psychological problems
> - ...
>
> ... and for the light ones:
> - teeth
> - visual problems
>
> ... it is not useful for diseases caused by:
> - malnutrition
> - intoxication or poisoning
> - injury from overload or trauma
>
> (Because these last three illnesses are not caused directly by a psychological cause.)

Note: When we have a disease from birth, we must look for the psychic shock during pregnancy, or trauma from our ancestors that we have received through our parents.

For this, there are therapists who take into account genealogy (only objective facts about ancestors, such as dates of birth, death, children, diseases, accidents, ... it isn't to consult the spirits of the dead).

How do we get sick?

Hamer was a doctor (he wasn't a psychologist nor psychiatrist), and therefore, was focused on material things; and he saw that, starting from a given moment, the body begins to show changes, the illness begins.

> Hamer discovered that the illness begins when we experience an emotional shock
> (apart from when it is produced by malnutrition, intoxication or lesion).

We can also call it 'big concern', or simply, 'a shock'.

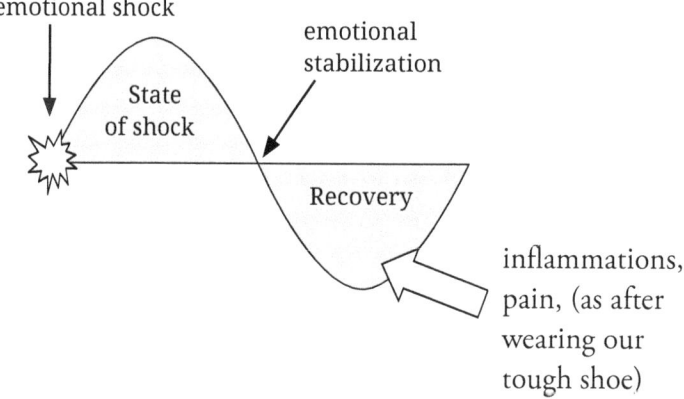

> Neither chemical products, nor the waves of cell phones directly produce cancer.
> There is not anything carcinogenic.
> But the waves or the chemical substances intoxicate us and weaken us, and, with a weak body, anything affects us more.

Usually, night rest is enough to repair what has been damaged during the day. But when this is not enough, because of the intensity and longevity of the emotional trauma, the body can't repair at night all that has been damaged during the day, and the body accumulates damage that, when repaired, causes very visible inflammation and pain.

How does the illness evolve?

The two phases of the illness

The typical symptoms of each period are:

Worry phase	Recovery phase
stress	fatigue and wellbeing
no appetite	good appetite
no rest at night	deep sleep
cold hands	warm hands

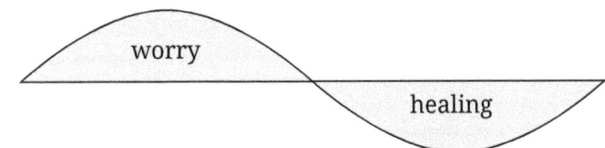

Frequently we realize that we are sick when we are already in the recovery phase.

In other words, illnesses like the following ones are only symptoms of recovery from a time of previous tension:

- ductal breast cancer
- lymphoma
- heart attack
- leukemia

Into these cases, it is necessary only to try not to relapse in the concern that caused them and to let the body perform the recovery by itself.

Other illnesses indicate that we are still in the phase of concern:

- breast cancer of mammary glands (the less common one)
- lung cancer
- prostate cancer
- pancreas cancer
- colon cancer
- osteoporosis

In these cases we have to solve the psychological cause to pass to the recovery phase.

In these cases Hamer warns us of the symptoms that we will have in the recovery phase, and so, we accept them better.

The psychological causes of each of the previous diseases are:

Symptom	Emotional Shock
breast cancer of mammary glands	worry for a loved one
lung cancer	fear to die
prostate cancer	not to feel oneself a man anymore
pancreas cancer	fights with other relatives
colon cancer	to feel that we have been offended
uterus cancer	worries related to reproduction or descendants

The whole list of illnesses, with their psychological causes and examples, can be found in the books of Dr. Hamer.

Inside some organs (stomach, bladder and uterus), cancers have different causes depending on their exact localization, and some cancer appear in the worry phase and others in the healing one.

The chronic illnesses

Illnesses become chronic because we take drugs that stop recovery.
For example:

Time when we have been decalcificating our bones.

We solve the psychological cause of our decalcification. Bones start to recalcify.

When bones recalcify, much pain arises.

We take an anti-inflammatory to ease the pain. This medicine interrupts the healing.

Bones cause no pain for a time (but they don't heal either).

When the body eliminates the medicine, repair continues and bone pain arises again.

We take another pill which again interrupts the healing process.

Until one day we learn about Hamer and we leave the body to repair completely once for all.

For example (previous page diagram):

We have passed a time in which we have had decalcification of the bones.

Now we enter the recovery time and they start to hurt us because recalcification begins.

We take anti-inflammatory drugs to stop the pain, but these stop recalcification.

When the body eliminates the medication, (because the medications are intoxicants and the body works to get rid of them), the recalcification of the bones restart and they begin to hurt us again.

In this way, we end up taking pills for the pain of bones all our life.

Chronic illnesses are also produced when we continually relapse into the concern.

Relapses before the recovery is completed

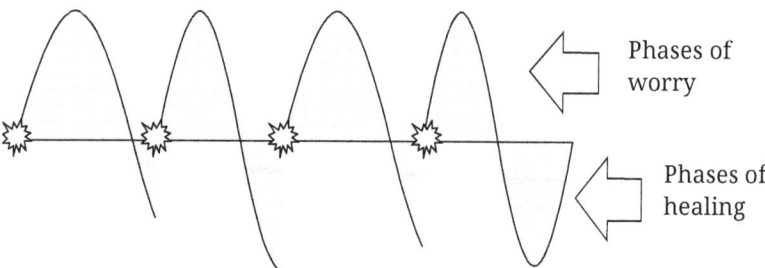

Even when recovery is complete, we can relapse another day, and have (for example) migraine attacks from time to time with greater or less intensity.

Relapses after recovery is complete

Relapses are something normal because we usually stumble twice against the same stone.

> Illness and healing are produced by our thinking.

Illness begins with an emotional shock and recovery begins when we overcome that shock and we liberate ourselves of the concern.

Hamer helps us to discover, for each illness, its psychological cause that we should solve or to avoid relapse. And he teaches us to let illness evolve until total recovery (in the serious cases it's necessary to control this evolution).

> What matters is not what happens to us,
> but how we take it.

The same fact can produce different consequences:

Fact: We have lost some money (we don't find where we put it).

Possibility 1: We think that it is our fault because "we have a poor memory", or because we "give little attention to what we do", etc.
Consequence: decalcification of bones.

Possibility 2: We think that somebody has stolen it from us and we feel as if he is trying to offend us in some way.
Consequence: colon cancer.

Possibility 3: I am able to see the good side of what happened. Or I don't see it and I have some bad days but then I forget the matter thinking that with health I'll work again and made more money.
Consequence: any illness.

Continually we have emotional shocks that are more or less serious. The sooner we solve them, the less they will damage our body and in less time we will repair the lesions.

> No external fact makes us ill.
> Only our inability to accept it creates the emotional shock that makes us ill.

CT

Depending on where a mark appears in the brain scan, and according to its size, experts know:

- In which organ is the problem and what concern has caused it.

- The 'size' of the concern: if it has been more or less intense and long.
- At what point of its evolution it is (at the beginning or already recovering).

In his books, Hamer explains where these marks appear in the brain CT and to what disease they correspond.

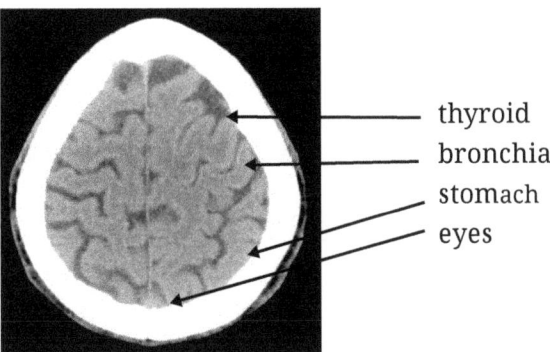

His books also explain what illness is caused by what worry or emotional shock (as explained above).

These marks are called "Hamer foci" in the literature. They have a target configuration.

Natural relapse at the middle of the healing phase

Halfway through the recovery period there is a natural relapse that must be known and prevented in severe cases.

This natural relapse has a different duration and symptoms for each disease.

The duration ranges from a few seconds to four hours.

This relapse may go unnoticed if the concern was mild and short-lived, or be more visible in the opposite case.

When the emotional shock was to feel the loss of all or part of what we considered 'our territory' (only in right-handed men), this relapse is a heart attack, which will be dangerous if it has been an intense feeling sustained for many months.

Heart attack is explained in a later chapter in detail.

How to get the original information of Dr. Hamer

Buying his books at Amici di Dirk publishers (in Spain). Phone: +34 952 59 59 10. E-mail: info@amici-di-dirk.com.

Browsing his web page at www.amici-di-dirk.com, where we can also buy his books.

Other means of popularization of his discoveries

Dr. Hamer's discoveries are called GNM, "new medicine" or "the five biological laws" by his most direct disciples.

They also receive many other names, with combinations of words or prefixes (or suffixes) such as: medicine, psycho, bio, biological, decoding, neuro, meta, total, new, ... and in general, all the books that talk about the mind-body connection – emotional origin of diseases.

Dr. Hamer's discoveries are not a therapy, just a diagnostic tool. For this reason, many different therapists use them for diagnosis and then apply their therapeutic specialty.

Internet web sites

Dr. Hamer approved sites:
- germanische-heilkunde.at (in German)
- neue-medizin.de (in German)
- free-news.org/htm/index-NP-GNM.htm (in Spanish)

Other web sites

- newmedicine.ca (from Canada, in English)
- 5lbtraining.it (in several languages)

- disease-is-different.com (with very clear and short videos)
- https://web.archive.org/web/20180809062712/www.alasanteglobale.com/tableau.html (in French, with an introduction to the "Hamer's tables")

> The best of Dr. Hamer's approach is that:
>
> - anyone can understand it
> - anyone can validate personally or in others
>
> Anyone of us can check the approach of Dr. Hamer when we see in his books how he spots correctly which is the emotional shock related to every illness.

And it warns us of the symptoms that we will have:

- sweating at night
- pain at the bones
- …

and so we receive them in a better mood.

Chapter 7

Putting Dr. Hamer's discoveries into perspective

The irrefutable evidence

Illness and psychological stress can be seen in the CT as a special form.

Nothing appears in the CT when there is neither illness nor concern, even in the most adverse circumstances.

If we smoke a lot, we will end up with the lungs full of tar and experience difficulties in breathing, but, if we don't fear dying, we won't develop lung cancer (and nothing will be seen in the CT).

Modern CT equipment filters these forms so nothing can be seen.

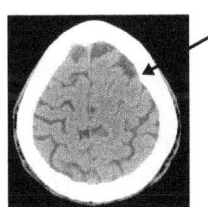

CT without form in the area of the lungs.
The lungs can be full of tar, but there is neither lung cancer nor fear of death.

When Dr. Hamer discovered these forms (target rings), his first reaction was to think it was a false image, a fault of the CT device.

With the help of the CT manufacturer's engineers, he learned to distinguish image faults from real forms (that can also be seen in MRI, or irrespective of the position or orientation of the patient in the CT device, etc.)

Hamer puts medicine 'upside down'

It is just as in life, where we discard our mistaken knowledge when we discover new truths.

As when the snake changes its skin, it leaves behind the dead skin that is of no more use.

Hamer's work has been known since the 1980's and its validity easily established.

Like the snake, thanks to Dr. Hamer discoveries doctors can leave erroneous knowledge behind.

Mainstream medicine is still valid, since Hamer's 5 biological laws don't explain everything, but his findings should cause these to be a reorientation in medical understanding.

Warning: Dr. Hamer wasn't God, he too made mistakes. Probably in diseases that are not very frequent and for which, therefore, he didn't have many cases to study. For example, he was very mistaken about retinal detachment.

On the different functions of medical practitioners and therapists

We ourselves, or with the help of someone, must come to a diagnosis:

What happens to me started with this and I'm here (still in tension)

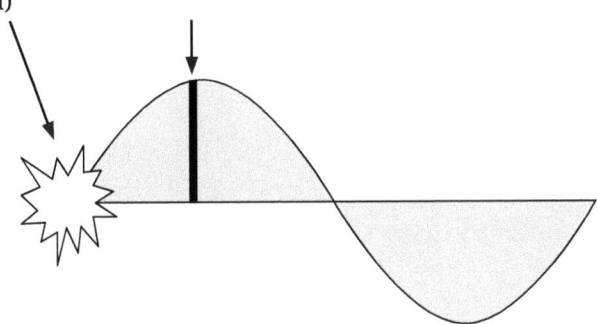

Or:

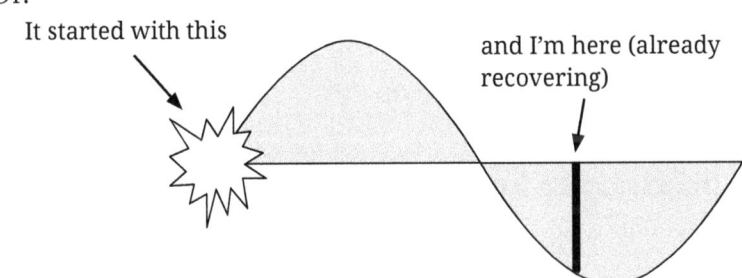

It started with this   and I'm here (already recovering)

In the first case, therapists are more useful because their therapies can help directly or indirectly the patient to overcome his concern quickly.

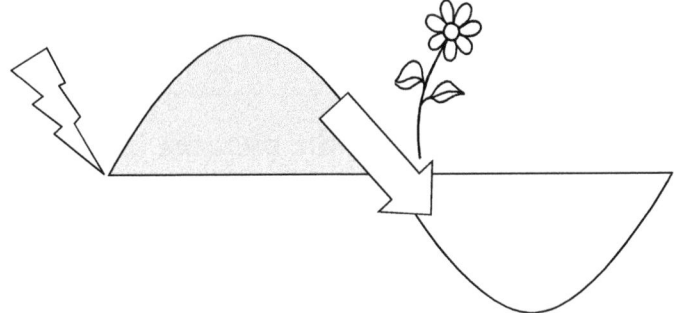

In the second, doctors are more useful, because in some cases it is necessary to use medicine to slow down the healing and make it less intense, or to carry out surgery.

In other words:

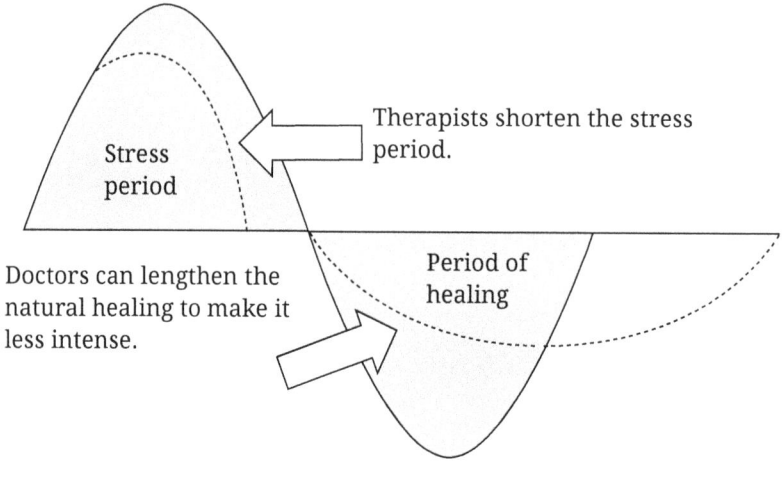

It is necessary to know about Hamer before we need to

Because when we are sick, we are not sufficiently balanced to understand it properly.

In addition, once we understand Hamer's ideas, we will see their validity corroborated in those around us, and this will give us a security more valuable than gold in understanding our own experiences, should we become ill.

Hamer's discoveries are not the panacea (the cure of all the ailments) because it is not a therapy

Hamer's discoveries only provide us with diagnoses.

It is very useful to have a true knowledge of our situation and what has caused it, but, once we know this, Hamer's discoveries don't provide us with a remedy: how to resolve our trauma and move into the recovery phase.

There is not a "Dr. Hamer's therapy" because the origin of the problem (and the solution) is mental, and the laws of Hamer only explain the functioning of the body. They are not tools to solve mental trauma.

In spite of their immense value, the five laws discovered by Hamer and the norms that develop them, don't cover all medical knowledge.

They don't explain all the functions of the body and they don't deal with the illnesses caused by non-psychic phenomena, like accidents, intoxication, overexertion or parasites.

The discoveries of Hamer are like a map that tells us (see the following page):

- Where we are.
- How we got where we are and how to get back.

We can leave by foot or by taking a taxi – having help if we can't solve our problems by ourselves.

If we take a taxi (go to a therapist) to leave from where we are, evidently the taxi driver should know the route (he should know of Hamer's discoveries). Otherwise, we will get lost together (like the chronically sick person who continues to take medication, and never fully recovers).

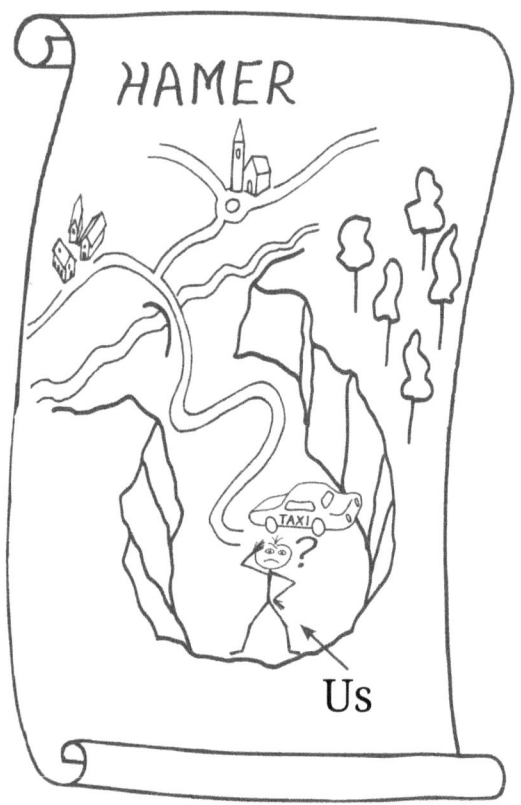

It's true that, although Hamer's discoveries are not a therapy, they helps us to avoid many problems simply by explaining; because common cancers such as the ductal breast cancer or the lymphoma only appear when the psychic shock is already overcome and the body only needs help to recover itself.

Chapter 8

Breast cancer and heart attack

Breast cancer

Ductal breast cancer ("invasive ductal carcinoma" or IDC) is the most common type of breast cancer (90% of cases). It's cancer of the milk ducts.

They carry the milk from the glands that produce it to the nipple.

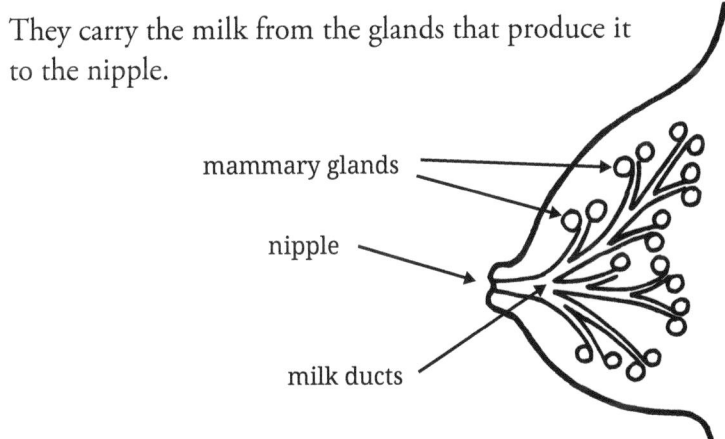

In right-handed women, cancer occurs in the right breast if they have felt traumatically separated from her husband, and in the left breast if they feel separated from their child (and vice versa for left-handed women).

The same thing happens in animals.

When cows are moved away from their calves, they suffer and contract mastitis, which is breast cancer in the milk ducts.

(Cattle ranchers draw their milk carefully so that it doesn't accumulate and doesn't hurt cows.)

When women suffer an emotional shock from the separation of a loved one, the milk ducts widen.

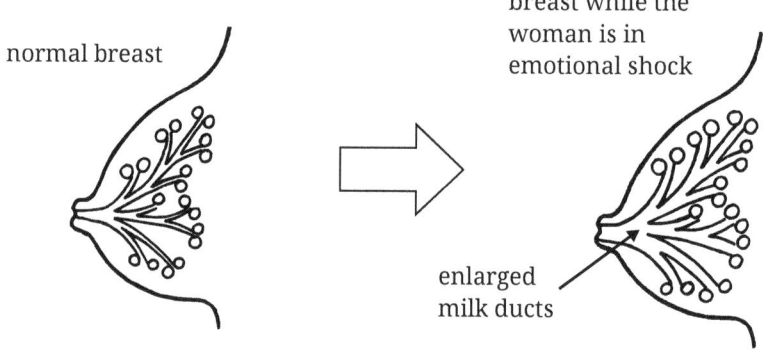

There are only two ways to widen a tube: thinning the walls or making cracks. It is this second way that happens.

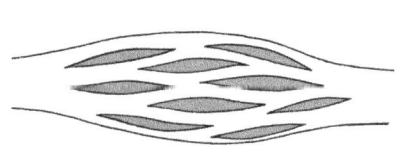

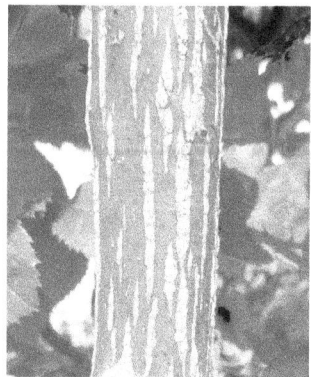

In trees, we can see cracks that form in the bark as they grow.

These cracks appear and enlarge while the woman **feels strongly separated from a loved one.**

But they don't produce any external symptoms or pain.

It is only from the moment when she overcomes this strong feeling of separation, that her body begins its repair work and the woman begins to feel the lumps in her chest.

These lumps are simply the healing of internal wounds in the milk ducts.

(As with any wound, when the cracks in the milk ducts heal, they become inflamed.)

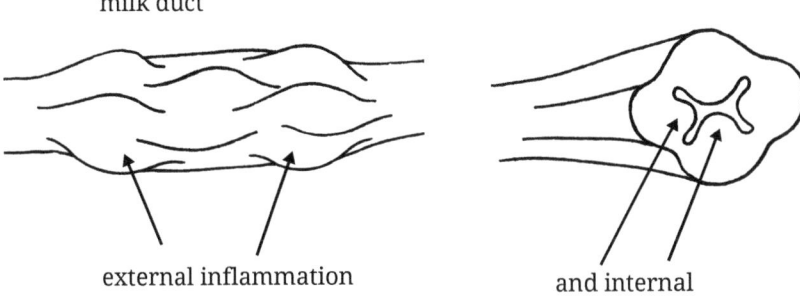

This inflammation, besides being felt like a lump from the outside, inside can clog milk ducts and cause pain.

The woman just has to let the body do its job: heal the wound. Normal life, normal diet, etc.

> The mental state is always the one that governs the course of the disease: overcoming the worry and not relapsing into it.

Lobular breast cancer
(10 % of breast cancers, "invasive lobular carcinoma", ILC)

The stones that appear in the breasts of some women are the end result of cancers of the "lobular" type (proliferation of the mammary glands) that they have inadvertently had.

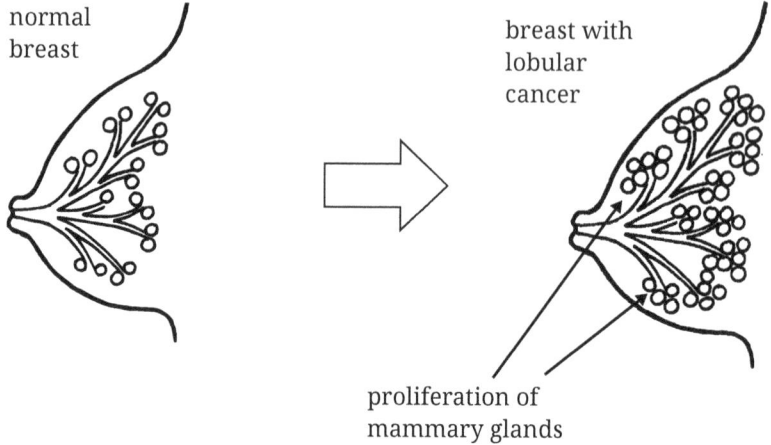

proliferation of mammary glands

The longer the time of suffering due to a loved one, the greater these calculi are.

(This doesn't mean that women who don't have stones in the breast don't love their families.)

As soon as she overcomes the concern, there are two possibilities:

1. The woman is not vaccinated against tuberculosis, so she **has** those bacteria which will eat the tumor and her breast will be back to the way it was before.
2. The woman is vaccinated against tuberculosis, so she **doesn't have** those bacteria and the tumor will turn into a stone, calculi.

If the woman has a mammogram during the stress phase, the tumor is growing. If she has it when she is healing, either we will not see anything (if she is vaccinated against tuberculosis) or we will see that a stone is being formed.

Heart attack (*)

Whenever we are healing from something, we have inflammation in the brain.

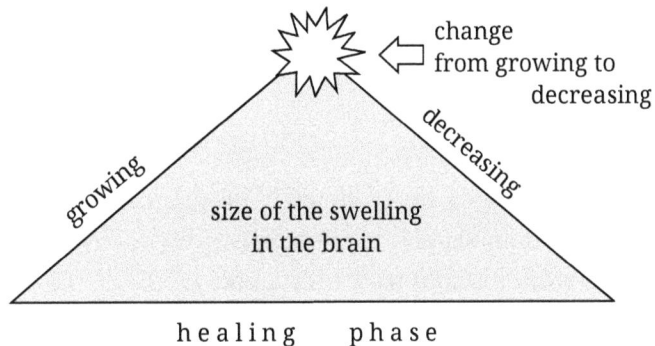

This inflammation increases until halfway through the healing phase and then decreases until it disappears. (Like the small inflammation of any wound when healing.)

The transition from growth to decline is externalized with certain different symptoms for each disease. And its duration depends on the disease (from a few seconds to four hours).

(This change is what we called "natural relapse" in chapter 6.)

When we feel a "loss of our territory" and we have struggled for a long time to recover it, this change is externally manifested as a heart attack.

This crisis can be fatal if we have fought intensely for several months.

(*) Heart attack and myocardial infarction are not the same. See details in Hamer's books.

> A Hamer expert, with the help of a patient's brain scanner, can help predict the severity and timing of a heart attack.

Joseph's case (real one)

Joseph has just had a heart attack. The doctors recommend he have surgery immediately. He, unexpectedly, leaves the hospital and goes to work his land with his tractor.

The doctors and family are worried for his life.

Luckily, his sister knows Dr. Hamer's approach and she calms them with the following explanation:

Her brother had a bad time because the bank wanted to evict him from his home. A few weeks ago he had convinced them to let him stay.

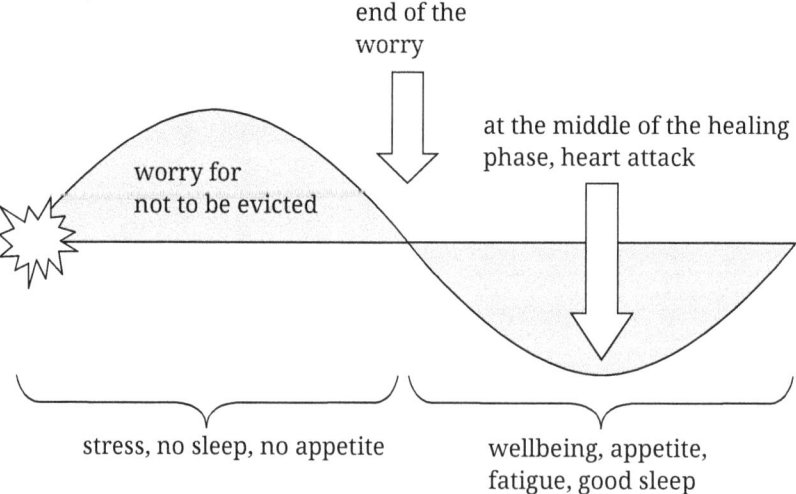

It was normal that he had a heart attack because that occurs halfway in the healing of a 'threat to our territory' concern.

It was normal that he went to work, because during our recovery, although we are tired, we are happy, we have a good appetite and we sleep well. And he didn't have any of this while struggling with the bank.

And when someone is well and happy, he is not willing to be operated on.

> **Cholesterol is not the cause of heart attacks nor tobacco the cause of lung cancer.**

(Though there's no excuse to continue eating bad food or smoking tobacco, both full of sugar and preservatives.)

Chapter 9

Therapeutic guide for the patient

> **Warning**
>
> Before we start taking more than one or two tablespoons of sea water a day, we should read and understand Dr. Hamer's approach.
>
> If we take more sea water, our body may start to heal with symptoms that, without knowing Dr. Hamer's approach, we can confuse with an illness.
>
> Besides sea water, also warmth, rest, a good meal, good company, anything that calms us can trigger the healing process.
>
> In an extreme case, anything can cause this healing, depending on personal circumstances:
>
> - A boy can begin to recover from being unfairly overlooked just by receiving an small prize, with symptoms that, if treated inappropriately, can be very detrimental to him.
>
> Therefore, it's urgent and important to know as soon as possible Dr. Hamer's approach.
>
> This book explains the general theory of both Hamer and the use of sea water.
>
> Health professionals who know these two theories are the best prepared to apply each of them.

We can ourselves do what this chapter explains or ask a professional for help (see later on "Where can we find help?").

In this chapter we will see the steps to follow, depending on the situation.

- Situation number 1: We are well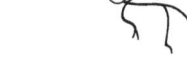

- Situation number 2: We are sick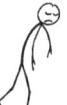

- For terminally ill people or emergency situations

> **First of all: we can decide whether to drink sea water or not**

After reading this book, we may have a hunch or feel whether sea water is for us or not.

Why feel or have this intuition? Aren't the reasons seen in the previous chapters sufficient?

Reason has its limits and it's not enough to guide our conduct.

We don't make life's important decisions (whom we marry, what we study, what profession we choose, etc.) using only reason.

> When we are calm, free from prejudice and desire, our body can help us to decide which alternative to choose, looking at the subtle body reactions that we have when we think about each option.
>
> We can also use it for daily decisions.
>
> Or to use intuition.

Natural things like the sun, fruit, sea water, ... are generally always beneficial.

But when we move from general to specific situations, we find cases in which natural things can harm us:

- The sun burns us if we expose ourselves too long when we have very white skin or when we climb a very high mountain.
- Fruits are good if we eat them outside of meals. If we eat them for dessert, they spoil our digestion (except for apples).
- We can wash our nose with undiluted sea water, but only from time to time. If we do so every day, we have to dilute it.

There are cases in which it is not advisable to take more than one or two tablespoons of sea water per day because it can trigger important healing processes which our body doesn't have sufficient energy to complete.

> It's like when we start works on a road and the money runs out before they are finished.
> In the end we are worse off than at the beginning, because the works are not finished and vehicle circulation is blocked.
> (We neither heal nor have the energy to stay alive.)

Besides, we are very complex beings. And there are some psychological circumstances, with several simultaneous concerns, where even Dr. Hamer dared not recommend the start of the healing process because of its unpredictable evolution. Sometimes it is better to gradually let go of the concern without resolving it completely.

> For added security, let's see a doctor who knows Hamer's approach.
>
> Looking at our brain scan, an expert can know how dangerous it is to start a major healing process.

> Sea water can help us during healing, but we, listening to our intuition, can come to know, better than anyone, whether we should begin this healing or not.

Situation number 1: We are well

Once we drink sea water every day, there are two possibilities:

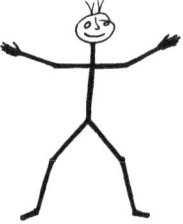

1. We don't feel any change if we were doing well before and our body was clean from the inside. We can continue to drink it, preventively.
2. We feel an improvement in our general condition. We feel better from all angles.

In this second case, if we feel better now, it's because before we were not so well. We have spent some time without our bodies functioning normally.

What does our body do all day apart from being active and happy?

Continually (and especially during the night), it repairs itself and recuperates.(*)

(*) Let's remember that every 7 years we renew all the cells of our body (except the nerves).

If our body has returned to normal functioning and we have significant damage to repair, within a few weeks the repair process and its troubles will begin.

> It's as if we're living next to a road blocked by an overflowing river.
>
> Since trucks don't flow, there is no noise or disturbance.
>
> What happens when the overflow ends and traffic restarts?
>
> Quickly a lot of trucks, more than usual, pass by and produce a lot of noise and vibrations: these are all the trucks that were waiting.
>
> When the road is not blocked, we don't notice the trucks because they only pass from time to time.
>
> Now that they all move one after the other, they are clearly audible.
>
> The same thing happens with the body:
>
> If it works normally, it makes repairs that go unnoticed.
>
> But if for a while it cannot make them, the work accumulates, and when it can finally do them, all the repairs are much more spectacular, and the disturbances much greater.

We will discover that we were not as well as we thought, because we had impending repairs. And, once the annoyances due to the repairs are over, we will recover a higher level of wellbeing and health.

Our body may have impending repairs for the following reasons:

- When we continually poison it with medication.
- When we don't nourish it sufficiently.
- When we don't give it rest during the day because of concerns or physical work and we don't sleep well at night.
- When there are other things that consume energy, such as dental infections or devitalized teeth (with "root canal" treatment), or when there are scars that continue to irritate the nervous system long after the end of an injury. All of these things take energy from organs that share the same meridian, and are treated with neural therapy (after any necessary tooth extraction). See *Dr. Adler's book* in the Bibliography.

Sea water helps us in the first two cases.

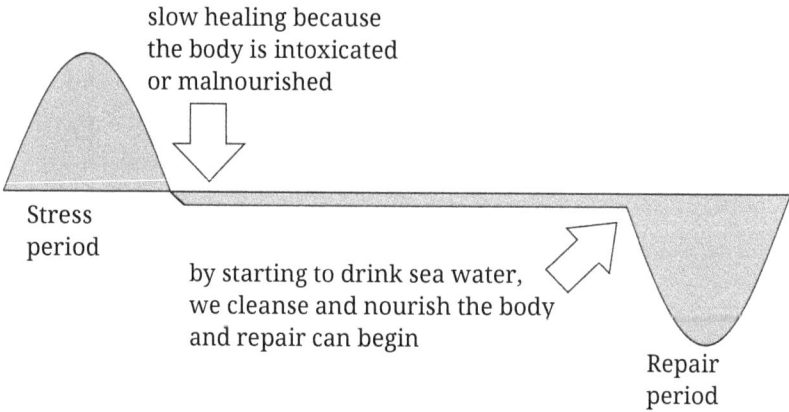

If after starting to drink sea water there is significant discomfort we can follow what is said next.

Situation number 2: We are sick

In this section we will see the two steps to follow:

1. To discover how we got sick and whether we're in the recovery period or still in the stress period.
2. To apply therapies or remedies to help the body do the impending repairs and avoid relapse into the concern that is causing our illness.

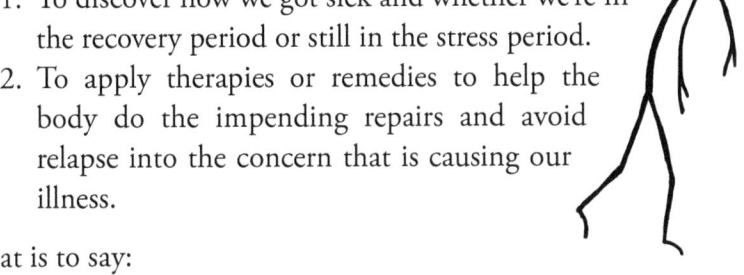

That is to say:

1) To discover what is the concern that caused my illness and to find out if I am still in a stress phase or already in the healing phase. (If it has no other origin such as: poisoning, accident, parasites or malnutrition.)

> Searching the illness in the "Hamer's tables" we find entries like:
>
> - Lung cancer: fear of death, desire to live.
> - Breast cancer: feeling painfully separated from her husband or child.
> - Decalcification, osteoporosis: feeling inferior to others in a certain aspect.
> - Etc.
>
> (The end of Chapter 6 explains how to obtain this information.)

> Sometimes the most visible symptoms of the illness start with the last emotional shock we experienced, but sometimes it's the opposite: they appear when we have just overcome the shock.
> So: leukemia, lymphoma, breast cancer and hemorrhoids appear right after we come out of a big concern.

97

> In these cases, our body was altered during the concern but we didn't feel anything.

In the tables we confirm what, perhaps, we already knew: what concern is the cause of the disease.

Thanks to them, we now know if we are in a stress or healing phase, because we know if we have resolved it or not.

In addition, we verify the symptoms in our body are those predicted in the tables:

Symptoms during the concern phase are:

- irritability, cold hands and feet, poor appetite, insomnia,
- ulcers with associated pain, angina pains, high blood pressure,...

Healing symptoms are:

- inflammation, tingling, redness, heat or fever,
- headache, muscle pain, bone pain,
- tranquility, warm hands and feet, good appetite, deep sleep, fatigue, low blood pressure,
- pus and hemorrhages (vaginal, anal, bloody sputum, ...) are cells that the body no longer needs, such as overripe oocytes or tumors that have become unnecessary.

The other way to find out the cause of the disease is by doing a brain scan (without contrast *), and asking for its analysis by a Hamer's expert.

(*) Contrast is a radioactive fluid that colors the image and is not useful for Hamer's analysis. Without contrast, the image is more real.

2) To apply therapies or remedies to help the body do repairs and avoid relapse into the concern that is causing my illness.

If we are still in the stress phase, sea water will relax our body, and so we will have more serenity to find the solution of the concern.

During this phase, we must not forget that our goal is to resolve the concern so that the body enters the healing phase.

In the next section, we mention some psychological work that we can do to resolve the concern.

Sea water will calm us down and can reduce the body's symptoms, but it doesn't resolve the concern.

If we don't resolve the concern, as soon as we stop drinking it, symptoms will return (for example constipation).

If we are already in the healing phase, sea water will help us to complete it faster and with a better general condition.

> In most cases, just living normally the body heals itself.

Remember that ductal breast cancer, lymphomas, bronchitis,... are just symptoms that appear during the healing phase.

We just have to continue our life and usual diet for the body to complete its healing.

Sea water will help us, but our body can also achieve the healing without it.

Sea water will not keep us from going through the symptoms of this stage and symptoms will go away on their own when the healing is over.

> Just as work trucks disappear with their noise and disturbance when they finish repairing the street.

While we are healing, we can use appropriate remedies but always remembering: that we will go 'forward' if we resolve the concern that caused the illness, or we will go 'backwards' if we relapse into it.

A complication to be avoided:

The most common complication is fluid retention. It can happen when we bring a sick person to the hospital and this fact makes him feel like 'a fish out of water'. This jeopardizes the success of the healing.

If the main cause of this fluid retention cannot be avoided, Hamer recommended various symptomatic treatments, one of which is an isotonic salt water bath.

As a diuretic, sea water, taken in any way, is very effective.

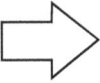 When the concern was intense and lasted for several months, Hamer recommended monitoring the healing process with frequent scanners.

It may be appropriate to take drugs (anti-inflammatories), which slow down the healing and lengthen it, but which prevent healing from exhausting the patient's energy. (Thus died the TB patients, see details in Appendix A.)

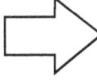 It is also necessary to slow down the healing when the size of the inflammations risks blocking bronchi and suffocating the patient.

(This occlusion is similar to that described on p.84 and 85.)

Instead of corticosteroids we can use other stimulants at hand (tea, coffee, cola), refresh the head of the patient as in the case explained in Chapter 13, or keep him active as much as possible.

Psychological aids to resolve the concern

Hamer helps us to find out what is happening to us and what concern caused it. This is the diagnosis.

If we are still concerned, we can use psychological therapies (such as EMDR, EFT, etc.), talk with a friend, or confess with a true priest[*].

> Speaking or writing about what hurts us is often enough to overcome the concern.

(*) A priest ordained prior to 1968. More information in ecomercado.es.

Acupuncture, homeopathy, Bach flowers, herbs, diets, etc. can also help us.

> A person's concern can depend a lot on his surroundings. Even if the patient is the one who finally directs his illness, in some cases it's preferable that psychological therapies involve family members.

To avoid relapse into this or other concerns, we should do more in-depth work, which is explained in the next chapter.

Sea water and cold on the head during healing

The more sea water we take, the faster and more intense the healing. The less we take, the longer the healing will take but it will be more bearable.

It doesn't matter if we take it diluted or undiluted, the effects are the same. We don't count the quantity of sea water we use for cooking because by heating it, it loses its properties.

> If the healing is too intense and causes us too much pain or inflammation, we may reduce the dose or stop taking it for a few days.

As we saw in the previous chapter, talking about the heart attack, every time we are healing from something we have a swelling in the brain (which doctors call "brain tumor").

It's this inflammation that produces the headache, and the bigger it is, the more intense the headache will be.

If we apply cold to the head, this pain will subside without interrupting the healing process.

> On the other hand, if we take anti-inflammatory drugs, the

headaches will stop but the body will also stop its healing until it eliminates them.

We can put a cold cloth or ice pack on the area of the head that is more hot and painful and avoid getting hot on the head. For example, we shouldn't expose our head to the sun or go to the sauna.

Other comments

Generally, the more serious the illness, the easier it is to find out the cause and the stage in which it is.
Small illnesses motivated by unimportant or very bearable concerns are more difficult to identify and resolve.

> It is easier to find and remove a horse from the garden than a rat, because we don't even know where the rat is.

To help with a patient's healing, it is very important that his trusted entourage (family, close friends) know Hamer's approach.

For terminally ill people or emergency situations

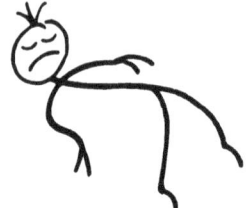

In these cases, sea water can lead to miracles and always improves the state of mind.

As René Quinton verified:

- With dogs that he bled completely (and that he made recover by injecting them with sea water).
- With dying people whom he saved in a few hours.

In these cases, the patient should be given a considerable amount of (isotonic) sea water.

In the case of hemorrhages IV injections are necessary because of their rapid action.

> Sea water (diluted) doesn't contain platelets, white and red blood cells, but it replaces their function until the body creates them again. Let's remember that the French medical vade-mecum said "It's possible to replace all the blood of an animal (...) without causing harm to it."
>
> Conventional "physiological serum" unbalances the organism[*], has contraindications, and in it white blood cells die. On the other hand, diluted sea water is neutral, in it live white blood cells and "it has no contraindications"[3].

In other terminal situations, intravenous injection is also the most appropriate way to give sea water, but if circumstances make it impossible, it can be given subcutaneously.

Always with improvement from the start.

(*) Conventional serum is acid (pH 5.5), while diluted sea water ("marine" serum) is neutral, with a pH of 7.2 like that of our body.

Let's look at two cases as examples:

> **A person in a hospital where medical use of sea water isn't recognized**
>
> As it is not possible to use IV or oral routes (if the patient is intubated), there remains only the cutaneous route (compresses of sea water on the head and other parts of the body), the ocular route, and maybe the anal route (with enemas of isotonic sea water). Even if the patient expels it some time later, he will still absorb something.

> **Terminally ill baby sent home to die after having undergone chemotherapy, radiotherapy, etc.**
>
> (We assume that we are in the best environment: a country where it is legal to inject sea water – not in the EU – and parents and family are receptive to treatment with sea water).
>
> Depending on the more or less critical state of the baby, injections and enemas are preferable to the oral route (using isotonic sea water).
>   We can also bathe him in lukewarm sea water, or apply sea water compresses on his head, but all this is superfluous if we have done what has been said before.
>   Instead, it will be much more beneficial if we hug him, skin against skin on the chest (*"kangaroo mother"*, *Mère kan-gourou*: cihr-irsc.gc.ca/f/46094.html).

Where can we find help?

In case the illness we want to overcome is not something simple like intoxication, and it has an emotional origin, we have to choose:

① Who will help us to identify the cause: **make the diagnosis** (a doctor or therapist who knows Hamer).
② Who will help us **to overcome the concern** (if we haven't overcome it yet).
③ Who will **help us during the healing** (especially if the concern lasted a long time and was intense and, therefore, we expect also an intense healing). See what is said in Chapter 7.

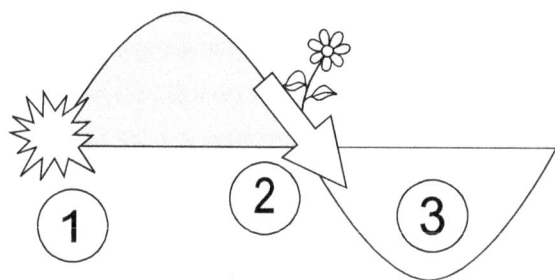

It can be the same person or it can be different ones.

The professional chosen for the diagnosis may have sufficient inter-personal skills to help us overcome the concern, or it may be better to undergo therapy.

Many doctors and therapists use Hamer's findings and give their therapies a variety of names, so it's important to know if they're really following Hamer's teachings (see information at the end of Chapter 6).

It's more difficult to find someone who, in addition, has experience in the medical use of sea water.

It's in Nicaragua where these findings are best combined, because Hamer is taught in the main universities and medical use of sea water is quite common.

> We can contact Santo Domingo Clinic (Tel: +505 22 22 25 98) where its director, Dr. Maria Teresa Ilari Valentí, promotes the medical use of sea water and Hamer in Nicaragua.
> There are also other addresses on the book's website.

Help! I've just had an emotional shock!

We have seen the importance of resolving concerns as soon as possible, so that the body has less work and the symptoms of healing go unnoticed.

How to resolve daily emotional shocks

Already Pythagoras, in his *Golden Verses*, told us how to do it:

> Doing an examination of conscience every night before going to bed. Acknowledging our mistakes and things we have done well. 'Making peace' mentally with everyone.
> As Paracelsus said: "Force yourself to desire the good of your greatest enemy. Your soul is a temple that should never be desecrated by hatred."

And may the last thought before we fall asleep be of absolute confidence that next day will be better.

> The last thought before we fall asleep, (and before we die), is very important because it decides how our dream will be. (This is why believers have always said that until the last moment we can repair a lifetime of mistakes – as narrated by Tolstoy's novel *The Death of Ivan Ilitch*.)

Maybe that's also why in the novel *1984* the Party tried to control people's thoughts until the last one, when dying.

> **Tips on what to do when something starts to upset us or relax when something has disturbed us**
>
> - To pray, to make the Sign of the Cross.
> - To urinate. Moms recommend to their children 'pee' after a fright. Perhaps because to urinate we must voluntarily relax the bladder sphincter. In this way, we force ourselves to relax so we can urinate.
> - To breathe deeply.

The night is the natural healing period from the stress of the day.

What better time to free ourselves from worry than when our body's natural rhythm takes us there?

> A hot shower or bath, like we do to babies before bedtime, is a big help. The Japanese often do.

If, every night, we repair the body damages resulting from the concerns of the day, the symptoms of the healing phase will go unnoticed.

> If night-time repairs have not been enough, we may devote one day a week to not working and to restoring peace wherever still exist some concern. (Believers call it "to keep holy the day of God – Sunday".)

Chapter 10

How to prevent emotional shocks

> Hamer tells us what is happening to us and why.
> But he neither tells us how to resolve the concern,
> nor what to do to avoid having it again.(*)

We have seen that many times, when we believe that we are sick, we are actually already healing (Wednesday).

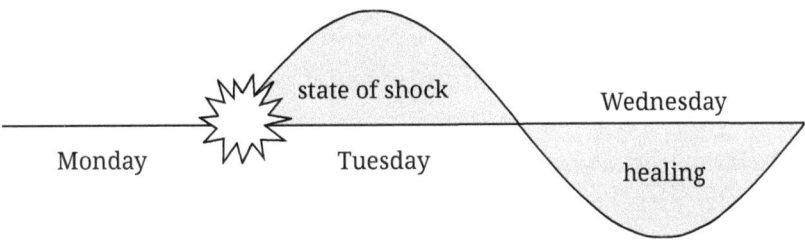

We have seen that Tuesday, when we are concerned, is the day we may need therapy to resolve the concern.

Hamer reminds us of what happened to us on Monday evening that started everything.

(*) An example of this was Dr. Hamer himself, who had great water retention due to his refugee status during the last years of his life.

> What can we do before to avoid the emotional shock of Monday evening?

We can see that we create difficulties for ourselves when we give **too much** importance:

To what we own (my house, my car, my jewels)
To our ideas (tastes, beliefs, etc.)
To what we want (I want this and I want it like this)
To what we think we are (English, lawyer)

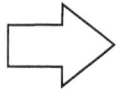 We can also feel as our own, and get sick from what happens to another person or to our favorite character in a novel.

So by taking what matters to us **too** seriously, we get upset when someone speaks badly of lawyers, or Englishmen, or what we like, or my car, house, etc.

Because we forget that we can change our car, house, profession or nationality and continue to be happy.

We can continue to be happy in any circumstance.

> During the day we can deceive ourselves and say that we are under stress because we have problems.
> But at night?
> At night, while sleeping, we cannot continue to think about our problems.
> Let's enjoy sleep and be the happiest in the world after doing what is explained in the previous chapter.

It's normal to be wrong and get sick. And to fall ill again for the same reason because we didn't learn the lesson.

It is impossible to always act perfectly, but we can always learn from our mistakes.

> We can learn by making mistakes, like children learning to walk: they fall and get up several times until they get it.

Thanks to Hamer, we know what we need to learn about each disease, because he tell us its origin.

In the case of the previously mentioned lost money:

- If the most important thing for me is to be otherwise (because I am not happy with myself), I will think that it's my fault if I lost it and my bones will decalcify.
- If the most important thing for me is to behave in an exemplary manner, without blemish, I will think that somebody, less perfect than me, stole it from me. I feel offended and so I'll make a colon cancer.

This will continue to happen to us until we learn that what we consider 'so important' is not.

> Real case: man with colon cancer. When asked if sometime he has been offended, he replied: "not just once, many!"

- I can try to be otherwise,
- I can try to behave perfectly,

but not be **obsessed** with it.

> The literal translation of "the Demon" in the Koran is "the obsessor" (*Sheitan*).
>
> He is who makes us take things too seriously: the good of Humanity, our prestige, our goods, etc.

And let's not use the knowledge that Hamer gives us to judge those who are sick:
- Because we are nobody to judge.
- Because another person's mistakes don't excuse mine ("I hit him because he insulted me.")

Recall that in the judgment scene of the Egyptian *Book of the Dead*, after death, the hearts of each of us are weighed individually.

Those weighing more than a feather are devoured by the crocodile who is attentively watching the needle of the scale.

What my neighbor's heart weighs won't make mine lighter.

(Our heart is heavy when it's filled with desires, fears, hatred, bitterness,...)

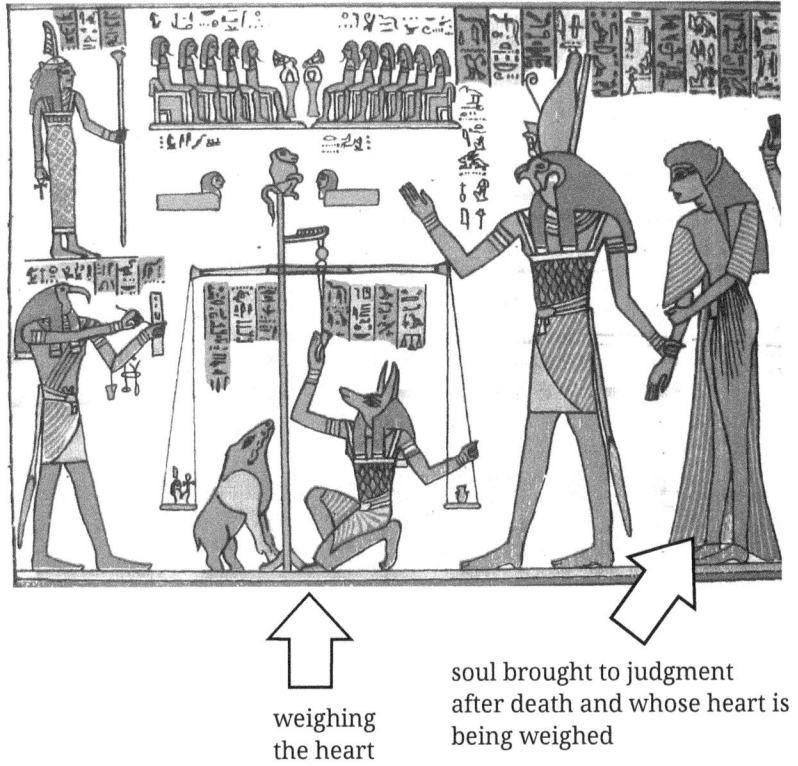

weighing the heart

soul brought to judgment after death and whose heart is being weighed

We must do things with care and attention, but without obsessing over what we do or the result.

- Because there is something to do at every moment, and if we are obsessed with a task, we will have a hard time leaving it and we will arrive late for the new task.
- Because often results happen by the confluence of many factors and we are just one of them.

> **Summary to avoid emotional shocks**
>
> - Let's do what we do with interest and care but without being obsessed with the task or the result. (Neither lazy nor obsessed)
> - If insurmountable setbacks arise, we must accept them as soon as possible and dedicate ourselves to something else.
>
> As Lole and Manuel say in their song *Todo es de color*: "hacer consuelo en todas las heridas" (*Everything has a color*: "to heal all wounds – psychic and in relations with others")
>
> In the same song they ask us to remember "beautiful things in life", which serve as support in times of difficulty.

> Behave like water, which is never obsessed: it doesn't want to take a particular shape and adapts to any container.
>
> And since it accepts everything, no one can hurt it, neither the sword nor the hammer.

Okay, I'm going to act without stubbornness or self-interest. But then, what do I do?

We are all different and have received natural gifts and weaknesses.

Our particular mission is to use our natural gifts (without pride, because we received them for free), avoiding as much as possible falling into our weaknesses. (Astrology can help us to know them.)

And, in general, we can devote ourselves:
To loving everyone (ourselves and our enemies *) to the utmost:

- with all our might
- with all our heart
- with all our intelligence

(Let us do, with joy, what we understand is best for everyone, including ourselves and our enemies.)
This is to keep the heart and the head together.

> Hitmen in films are an example of people who don't seek the good of all.(**)

It is easy to be wrong and dedicate ourselves to something which, as we learn more, we see produces the opposite effect to our intention.

In this case, we rectify it as soon as possible, and without further remorse, we dedicate ourselves to something else. ("The father makes a greater feast for the returning prodigal son, than for the faithful son." Luke 15:11).

Doesn't life lose its charm if we don't fight, if we don't suffer and we don't rejoice?

Feeling pain is useful because it warns us that we have had an injury that we need to treat.

(*) "Everyone who hates his brother is a murderer" I S. John 3:15, "Whoever is angry with his brother is liable to judgment" Matthew 5:22. Real farewell statement from a mother to her son departing for the 1936 war in Spain: "Don't hate enemies".

(**) In the fabulous film *Once Upon a Time in the West*, Morton is playing cards with bandits whom he wants to convince to kill their boss. Instead of cards, he puts 100 dollar bank notes on the table. A bandit asks him: "How do we play to this game?" Morton replies: "It's very easy, just use your head". (Because to murder someone for money we can only use the head, the heart refuses.)

We can accept the pain and forget it soon, like children who fall to the ground playing and get hurt, and are comforted by their mother. In a moment they forget their injury, their pain, and continue playing.

Or we can bear the pain with suffering. Suffering is another way to learn. Slower. Like the path on the left in *Ascent of Mount Carmel* of Saint John of the Cross.

When we are doing very delicate things or things that require a lot of effort, interests and fears disturb us.

The best artists, best judokas, best archers know that in the most important moments they have to put aside their interests and fears.

When we adults propose to our adolescent children:

- that they strive to own a home and car
- and then strive to keep them

they completely refuse.

Because they remember that, beyond the struggle, satisfaction and suffering that is offered to them, life has wonderful things.

And they claim them.

Chapter 11

Doctor - patient relation

Nobody can predict the future

All prognoses of an illness, though based on sound diagnostic theories such as Hamer's laws, are limited because they are the result of one doctor's experience and knowledge and cannot encompass all possible variables: medication, diet, environment, relapses in emotional trauma, etc.

This way, when we receive an unfavorable diagnosis such as:

> "You won't recover your vision because you have suffered from too many relapses"

we should remember the above-mentioned and add mentally (if the doctor doesn't say it):

> "It is possible that there is another doctor with other experiences and knowledge who can cure us".

Each therapy is ideally suited to a particular malady

Each treatment or remedy is more appropriate for some things than for others.

If we apply an inappropriate remedy, we lose the time that we could have used in applying a more appropriate remedy.

For example: If we beak an arm, drinking sea water will be beneficial but, if we don't go to the doctor to put the arm in plaster, it will not heal well.

Or it can become a perpetual crutch compensating for something that is wrong in another part of the body.

For example:

- Sea water is a good laxative but it doesn't cure the origin of the problem. We can take sea water for constipation, but should seek to find the cause and then cure it permanently.
- Similarly, we shouldn't use the fact that sea water helps with hangovers as an excuse to continue getting drunk.

A treatment or remedy can exhaust a patient's energy

We can assimilate stimuli up to a certain level. If that level is exceeded, we either protect ourselves from them or they harm us.

Examples:

- There are people living the whole day under the sun, but for those with a very fair skin, problems will result unless they take precautions to cover themselves.
- There are people that can look at the sun directly, but most of us cannot, and to do so causes ocular lesions.
- There are shamans that use hallucinogenic drugs daily, drugs which cause others to suffer insanity.

We are responsible for what happens to us

However, we should not use this fact as a moral judgment on the sick person or ourselves.

> As Jesus passed by, he saw a man who was blind from birth. His disciples asked him saying: "Master, who did sin, this man or his parents, that he was born blind?" Jesus answered: "Neither has this man sinned nor his parents; but that the works of God should be made manifest in him." (John 9).

Jesus avoids judging, and he helps the disciples to transfer their attention from the simplistic idea: 'we have found the cause, we have found the **culprit**'(*), to a '**for what** reason', complex and thought-provoking.

(Those 'why' are negative, those 'what for' are positive. Jesus invites us to look at the positive aspect in everything.)

Instead of punishing ourselves with a 'why did this happen to me', we can think: 'for what purpose did this happen to me', 'what can this teach me?' And Hamer shows us it very clearly in his books.

The best therapy is the one that teaches us how to prevent ourselves falling sick again

> It's the same as when we take our car to the garage, to change some worn out tires. A good mechanic will tell us: "I will change the tires, but if you don't align the steering, the new tires will wear out very quickly".

If we learn how to prevent illness, we avoid being dependent:

- on a doctor, therapy, medication, product or rite which transforms us into a chronically sick person
- on an unpredictable destiny in the form of 'multiple causes'

> It's not an evil being that wore out the tires, neither is it bad luck. It's because the steering wasn't properly aligned.

(*) In some societies (African tribes, companies in Japan), when somebody gets sick or makes an error, the whole community meets to confess how everyone believes that he or she could collaborate to this fact. (See "Hansei" in www.ki-rainet.com, about this tradition in Japanese companies.)

Therefore, if doctors understand the cause of illness, results won't be dependent on a blind destiny.

This understanding will also free them from therapies that were only successful because they were applied when the patient was already in the recovery phase.

> Any therapy or remedy, that it is applied when the patient is already in the curing phase (he or she has leukemia, ductal breast cancer, etc.), will be successful. (The exception is when this therapy interrupts the recovery by poisoning the body or weakening it, or when the patient relapses into the mental trauma that caused the sickness in the first place.) The same happened to Quinton when he applied sea water to people who were sick with cancer (see Appendix A: "Scientific basis").

We can help the body in excess

If we've had an accident and broken a leg, once the plaster comes off, we attend physiotherapy, where we are helped to recover movement in the leg.

At the beginning, the physiotherapists help us a lot, because we can hardly stand. Gradually we need less help, until we can stand and walk unassisted.

If instead of this, we were given excessive help (in the form of a wheel chair instead of doing physiotherapy), we wouldn't do the exercises necessary to recover and would remain wheelchair bound.

The same happens in other parts of the body.

The body doesn't always perform equally. We are not machines. There are days that we are more tired, other less, some days we see a bit better, others a bit worse, etc.

(We can see badly because a temporary deformation of the eye, because the muscles that orient it are continuously stressed.)

If the day that we see a bit worse we wear some lenses, we will see well but... when the stress of the eye muscles disappears and the eye tends to restore its shape, we will see worse with the lenses and the eye will stop its recovery. The eye will adapt to the 'help'.

If on another day when we see a bit worse, we do the same thing, this results in ever stronger lenses being needed for normal vision.

The same thing can happen with blood pressure, hearing, the kidneys, the heart, the thyroid, etc.

> Before embarking on a remedy or a therapy, we must understand, as much as we can, what is happening to us. Because often, the malady is only temporary and easily corrected by the body itself.

Are we falling into the 'halo' effect?

When a person attracts us by a certain feature (beauty, power, intelligence, ...), we tend to excuse his other imperfections.

When this happens in a relationship between a man and a woman, we say 'he is in love': he sees one aspect of the woman but is totally blind in regard to the other aspects.

This can happen in any relationship: fathers and sons, teachers and students, men and women, or doctors and patients.

We can be amazed by the beauty of a clinic, by a brilliant diagnosis and not see that the advice we receive isn't what suits us best.

And on the contrary, an aspect that we don't like in a person can make us deaf to his good advice.

Chapter 12

Medical use of sea water in Nicaragua

Since 2003, sea water has been used medicinally and nutritionally in Nicaragua. Fifty doctors and therapists prescribe it and they distribute 5,000 liters of sea water monthly (mainly in Managua and the surrounding area).

Nicaragua is where sea water is used more extensively in mainstream medicine and where there is a well-established system of distribution.

To achieve this, entities of all type collaborate: government ministries, universities, city councils, associations, different orders and religious congregations, companies, foundations and doctors, therapists and volunteers.

These entities collaborate freely, and their collaboration ensures that everyone can receive it free.

The universities analyze the water and they instruct doctors on its medicinal use; the government support is cross party, unaffected by changes in leadership; the city council of Managua collaborates over the transport, business provides resources; diverse orders and religious congregations give their facilities and vehicles for distribution; the foundations support financially when it is necessary, and the associations seek to educate and inform the populace about the benefits of sea water.

And everything is moved by the hearts of all those who participate in these entities and of doctors, therapists, volunteers, sick and other users who have learned how to see the benefits of sea water.

> Since 2009, the works of Dr. Hamer are taught in the main universities of the country. In this way, illness is better understood, along with a powerful remedy.

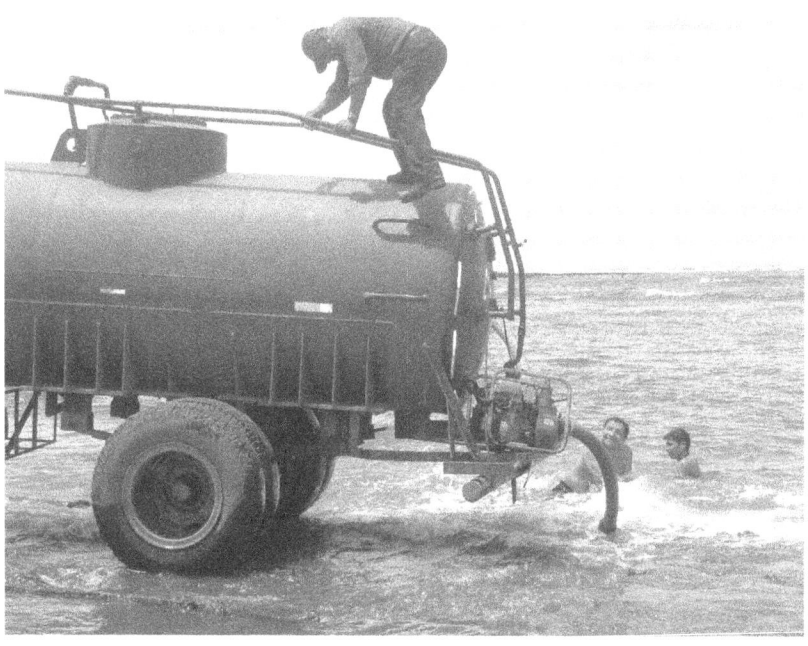

Sea water is collected at the Pacific's beach nearest to Managua with a truck tanker that loads the water while parked on some rocks (the water is not crystalline).

> The water is not treated in any way.
> Biochemical analyses have always certified it is free of any pathogen.

Next is presented a summary of the survey carried out by the author in February of 2009 to patients treated with sea water.

(It can be downloaded complete from the book's web. In Spanish).

Summary of the survey

The survey was carried out in public and private clinics of Managua thanks to the invitation of Dr. Mª Teresa Ilari, head of the Clinic St. Domingo (which belongs to the Jesuits), main distribution center, and thanks to Sis. Julie Marciacq who organized the interviews efficiently.

The diet of the interviewed patients is based on rice with beans, meat, milky products and some vegetables.

They often drink "frescos", made with fruit juice and sugar, and sugary drinks. They eat very few vegetables.

Results

The patients interviewed use or have used sea water as a medicine, alone or in combination with other medical treatments or conventional medicines.

The patients drink either undiluted sea water, sea water diluted with fresh water, or sea water diluted with fruit juice. Sometimes they use it as an ingredient in lemonades (natural ones), and they also use it for cooking.

The form and times of taking it vary considerably, and they take between 150 and 500 ml daily.

The patients report an improvement of their wellbeing and of their energy, a reduction in the need for conventional medications, a reduction in the time taken to become well, better final state of recovery or complete healing of the illness.

They also report solution to ailments that conventional medicine considers irreversible (such as primary cataracts).

> One of the patients reported that she found her neighbor's daughter being veiled and expected her death at any moment. She applied sea water with cotton to her lips (as she couldn't drink anything).

She sucked it with growing strength. Later on, she gave her sea water with a teaspoon. She survived and continues well.

One of the therapists who prescribes sea water related that his grandmother was already using sea water medicinally in Colon, on the Atlantic coast of Panama, at the beginning of 20th century.

Listing of treated affections

(A brief explanation of each case can be seen in the complete report in the book's web.)

Acne	Alcohol (addiction or hangover)	Allergies
Alopecia	Alzheimer (senile insanity)	Anemia
Arthritis	Bronchial asthma	Burns
Cataracts	Cerebral stroke	Cholesterol
Circulatory system	Cirrhosis hepatic	Colitis
Colon inflamed	Constipation	Cramps in the legs
Cysts	Deafness	Decay (prevention)
Depression	Dermatitis	Diabetes
Diabetic Ulcers	Fatigue, low energy	Fatty liver
Flu	Fungi	Gall bladder

Gastritis	Glaucoma	Goiter (thyroid)
Headache	Heart Ischemia	Heart problems
Hemiplegia	Hemorrhage	Hemorrhoids
Herpes Zoster	Hypertension	Infected wounds
Insomnia	Itching	Kidneys
Knees	Lupus	Malaria
Malnutrition	Mange	Migraine
Narrow excrements	Nervous asthma	Neuropathies
Obesity	Osteoarthritis	Osteoporosis
Pain at joints	Pain at the calf	Pain in plant of the feet
Pain in rump and knees	Pancreatitis	Paralysis in legs, arms, hand
Parasites	Peripheral Nerves	Polyps in intestine
Prostate	Psoriasis	Psychosomatic problems
Rheumatisms	Satiety	Scaring of wounds
Scleroderma	Sclerosis	Sinusitis
Skin diseases	Stomach	Stomach pain
Stomach ulcers	Strain (pulled muscle)	Stress
Swelling of arms	Trembling mouth or limbs	Varicose Ulcers

Dr. Ilari:

"I treat cancer cases from the perspective of Dr. Hamer (...) Patients are cured of their ailments without the need for medication (...) But as a therapeutic tool (...) sea water is for me the first restorative element of health."

Magazine *Dsalud.com* October 2012.

Chapter 13

A case with initially 'bad results'

Initially, Maria felt sea water wasn't good for her,
but, thanks to knowing Dr. Hamer's approach,
she realized what was happening.
It allowed her body to complete its cure
and it reached a superior level of health.(*)

Maria, why did you begin to drink sea water?
I had already read something on the internet about how good it was, and that it cured many illnesses, and I wanted to try it but I didn't know either where to go nor where to contact people who could help me. Then I went to a talk about Hamer and sea water and I decided to try it. *(The weekly talks at the Plural-21 association in Barcelona).*

I began to drink *(six months ago)*, a measure of sea water with three more measures of fresh water, twice a day: in the morning and in the afternoon, a glass of 250 ml. A year and half ago I had cancer and I was treated with radiotherapy. I discovered my liver and kidney function was badly impaired. This is one of the side effects of the whole illness. I felt like a weight, behind the kidneys,

---

(*) If she hadn't known about Dr. Hamer's theories, she wouldn't have been able to understand the effect of sea water, and would have lost the benefit of this positive response.

and a pain that extended forward.

Then, after drinking the sea water, I realized that the pain that had extended forward had disappeared. I was livelier and stronger. It was not a very fast change, but little by little, little by little I began to feel better.

But I had an adverse reaction two weeks later. It was like a strong, strong, strong flu, with a lot of pain in my bones, widespread, as if there was an inner inflammation in the bones, and also a very severe headache. I also developed a cyst on my right wrist *(right arm, operated ganglion of the left arm)*.

I got scared a little because this reaction was severe, I felt bad and I thought that sea water wasn't good for me. Then I remembered the explanations of Dr. Hamer and I realized that this was normal, that I was healing, and decided to continue. According to Hamer, my symptoms corresponded to a recalcification of the bones, after a previous decalcification caused by a poor self-esteem, and yes, it corresponded because I have always had low self-esteem.

For a week the pain was getting stronger and I stopped drinking sea water for three days because the reaction was too strong.

On the fourth day I took it again. The pains were decreasing and in a week they ended.

During the six first days I had a bad headache, with a lot of heat in the head, in the brain area, as if I had fever but I didn't.

Where at the head?

It was at the top, in both sides. It was a very severe pain. Then I put a cabbage leaf in the refrigerator for a while, after that I put it on my head, and it absorbed the heat from the brain.

After several days, I resumed drinking sea water but at a lower dose, because I realized that I was very sensitive to sea water.

I stopped eating whilst I had the flu symptoms – headache, aching bones, aching all over. I could not sleep well, I got up three or four times each night and I also woke up with headache, I ate very little.

My hands were hot and my head felt swollen with heat coming from my bones.

It was like suffering from bad influenza. I wanted to stay in bed; I didn't want to do anything, simply rest. I was happy, but if I hadn't known of Hamer, I would have been very worried about my condition. As I knew it was a healing reaction, I took it more calmly.

> This case is an example of how, drinking a significant quantity of sea water (more than one or two spoonfuls daily), can start a process of bodily recovery that must not be confused with the onset of a new illness.
>
> In this case, Maria, besides having the cerebral tumor that we all have in any recovery, also developed leukemia as part of her recovery from decalcification.
>
> Thanks to knowing Hamer, she understood correctly what was happening to her, and continued taking sea water.

Chapter 14

Veterinary use of sea water

The application of sea water in animals is the same as in humans and has the following benefits:

1. It helps them grow better and healthier.
2. It serves to cure diseases.

Regarding the first, there are experiences in Nicaragua such as:

> "The Union of Farmers and Ranchers of Nicaragua has started to experiment with sea water in their cattle. Its use has shown nutritional benefits since they fatten faster and they get sick less than those not treated with the liquid." (*El Nuevo Diario*, March 15, 2006).
>
> See also those reported at the end of the survey of patients treated with sea water in Nicaragua on the book's website. They refer to chickens, cows, horses ...

The fundamental difference between humans and animals is that the illnesses that these suffer from are always the result of material causes.

Our body feels as real all that we think or imagine, while animals feel as real only material facts.

> That is to say, a person can develop liver cancer because he is worried about his economic status, even though he might never actually go hungry.
>
> Whereas an animal will only develop a liver cancer if he has genuine periods of starvation interspersed with periods of satiety.
>
> Grief for a lost puppy may bring about breast cancer in a female dog, whereas a woman can develop the same condition by worrying about the health of a distant cousin's son.

Sea water can be administered to the animals in the same way as to humans, but it is easier to employ bathing, subcutaneous injections, or simply sea water mixed with the animal's food.

If the animal is injected, he will lay for a while. The more water we inject, the more time he will remain lying.

> If we inject sea water without dilution, we must leave fresh water for the animal, because it will feel thirsty and it will drink three times the quantity that has been injected.
>
> We must always leave fresh water near the animal so that it can drink and compensate for the sea water that we can inject or give it with food.
>
> (If we inject it with undiluted sea water and don't let it drink fresh water, he will die of thirst).

In the food or broth, we add one third part of sea water. If we put more, it will be salty and it will make the animal thirsty, but it will recover more quickly.

Differences in animal physiology that make sea water administration simple

Animals don't have the skin sensitivity that we humans do. So, when we inject them subcutaneously without dilution, it doesn't cause problems. They don't show irritation or pain.

They don't have fear of the injections, instinctive in humans.

There are cases that seem to indicate that they perceive when they need it:

- A sick cat that was offered two bowls with water, one of them with diluted sea water, drank from both.
- A cat cured of a urine infection with sea water injections, when she saw the syringe again, far from escaping, she rubbed against it.
- A dog that, once cured, refused to receive more injections.

For general ailments, we inject the animal in the nape of the neck. This way it is more difficult for the animal to bite us. (See Appendix B: "How to give subcutaneous injections").

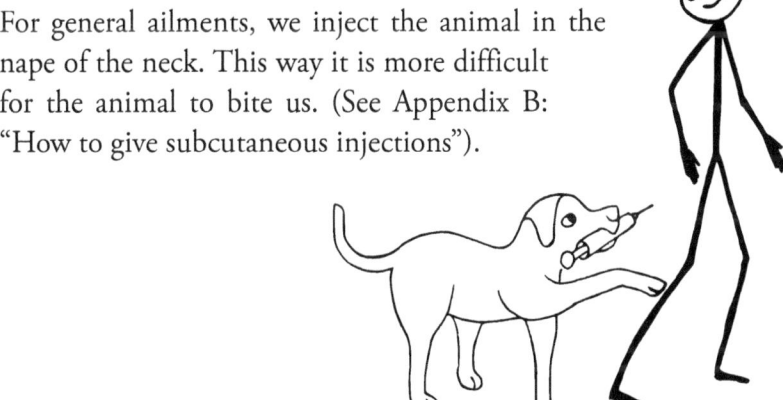

For localized ailments, we can inject them in the affected area, although sea water taken orally is equally effective.

Case of dog given up for dead

Name: Uma, golden retriever, 6 year-old.

Since she was two, she has had several tumors (breast, neck, armpit, paws) and she received four chemotherapy sessions.

She has never been in heat because she was sterilized after the first tumor.

For 3 years she took thyroid hormone (175 micrograms every morning and night), because she began not to move and to be inactive the whole day.

7 months ago, they removed a new tumor from among the fingers of her right rear paw. Then she had 3 months receiving chemotherapy every 15 days.

Two months ago, she stopped eating for 5 or 6 days. After tests, they diagnosed inflammation of the jaw and in the right side of the mouth. The inflammation oppressed her optic nerve with risk of her becoming blind.

She found it difficult to get up, and even experienced sudden paralysis while walking.

They administered cortisone. In a few days, the inflammation disappeared and she ate again. But then she stopped eating again (she even rejected a cookie!). In a few hours, the inflammation was back, along with dribbles, afterwards blood dribbles. She was very ill and she found it difficult to move. She even found it difficult to drink what was offered with the hand.

The cortisone treatment ceased and the dog sought solace in dark corners.

> "She didn't drink, we gave her something to drink but she could not open her mouth for anything. Besides that, she was all inflamed and her eye was being pushed out."

The veterinarian suggested to the owners to put her down.

Instead of that, the owners decided to inject her with sea water.

The critical time

They administered her subcutaneous injections of 10 ml of sea water at the neck. They injected undiluted, untreated, unfiltered sea water.

After the first shot she lay down completely for 15 minutes (this is a normal reaction).

> "After the first injection was assimilated she asked for more. After the second one, I noticed that it was doing her good. At the third one, I found she was more relaxed.
>
> But I didn't begin to be sure she was well until the next day in the afternoon when got up to drink and she seemed better.
>
> The dog's energy was very different. Before giving the first injection, she was dying. When I injected her with the sea water she began to react."

After each injection, the reaction was the same: she was prone for a while.

She didn't reject the injections.

Later, the same night, she was administered an injection of 50 ml.

The inflammation symptoms lasted until the following day but she had already got up to drink. (*Because she was injected with undiluted sea water, it made her thirsty and she drank three times the injected quantity, but of fresh water*).

They continued administering her injections of 40 ml for one week, one in the morning and another at night.

The dog recovered her normal behavior, even more vital than before, because now she chased rabbits, something never seen before.

They also gave her sea water with chicken broth. The prepared chicken broth was allowed to cool (until lower than 111 °F), sea water added and then given to the dog.

After a week of injections, the dog refused injections and she was given the sea water in her food: mixed with the food to soften it and making it less difficult for her to chew it. The dog first drank the water and afterwards the food. (400 ml daily of sea water without dilution). They put it also in the water for drinking (10% sea water and the rest fresh water).

She began to have diarrhea *(because she was taking too much sea water)* but that ceased after two days when the dose was reduced solely to her drinking water.

They reduced her dose of thyroid hormone to 150 µg.

A month later, they stopped giving her the hormone. Far from harming the dog, every day she was better, thinner.

> "The dog is better every day. She was always apathetic and now (6 years old) she asks to play with us, she asks to do things."

Now

> "Uma is jumping, with very good health, she is very lively. Before, she was a 'carpet' dog. She spent all day lying down, she didn't move and she didn't have dynamism. And now she is getting normal progressively. She moves more, she wants to play, and she has vitality. What she lacked before was vitality."

> "20 days ago I stopped giving her sea water, but now she is drinking it again because we've been putting it into her drinking water for the last four days."

> "Now we don't give her any medication and she is better and better every day. She is even losing weight. She is becoming a normal dog, having spent many years of abnormality."

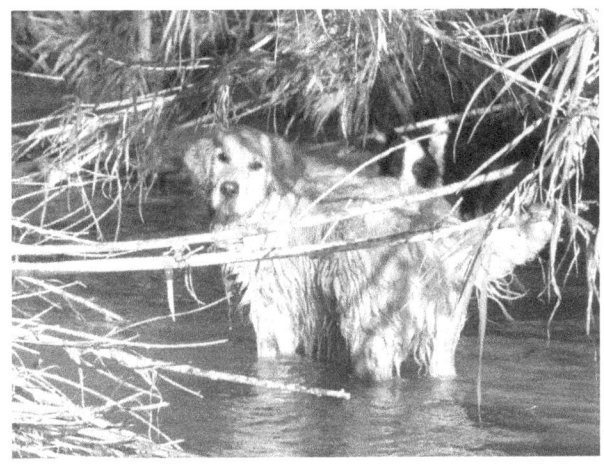

* * *

A video of the dog's condition, 3 months after the critical night, can be seen in the book's web page (it lasts only 5 seconds). The video shows her digging the earth, as any healthy dog does.

> In this case, sea water produced a spectacular result because the animal was only intoxicated.
>
> When the cause of the illness is a psychic trauma, sea water is only a help.
>
> Things that determine the course of the illness are:
> 1. a correct understanding of what is happening, according to Hamer's discoveries
> 2. the resolution of the psychic trauma that caused the illness
> 3. the prevention of relapse into psychic trauma.
>
> If 1, 2 & 3 are successful, a total cure should ensue.

Appendix A

Scientific basis

Extracellular matrix

The principle of medical application of sea water is the biological law that Quinton called "of the General Constant".[2]

Quinton states in his law that the sea was created at 111 °F, with 7.2 grams of salt per liter, and that cells of animals function optimally when they are in these conditions.(*)

He also states that the fluid which bathes all the cells of our body (the extracellular matrix), is sea water in its original composition (with only 9 grams of salts per liter).(**)

> This internal liquid or medium, due to its continuous exchange with the blood, has the same composition as the blood serum (without its organic components).
>
> The internal composition of cells is completely different.

(*) The importance of temperature for the better functioning of cells explains the benefits of all therapies that use heat: saunas, hot water baths that Japanese people take frequently, native "temascales", fever, etc.
(**) It is because of the universal deluge that the sea suddenly changed its concentration of salts per liter (creationscience.com).

Quinton demonstrated his theory by experiments on dogs – carried out again recently in France and Spain[*].

> He began by injecting into a dog weighing 10 kg, 10.4 liters **in 12 hours**. Its kidneys made 60 times more urine than they normally do. (9.4 kg of urine in 12 hours against 150 g normally).[2]
>
> And injecting 3.5 liters into a 5 kg dog, in an hour and a half, without giving the kidneys time to eliminate the liquid. "Initially, kidney elimination decreases. When the injection is finished, renal elimination accelerates. (…) On the eleventh day it's fully recovered and with extreme joy. Its weight returned to 5 kg."[2]
>
> And without permanent damage to kidneys, since in another case, he made a **total bleeding** (425 g) in 4 minutes to a 10 kg dog, and a posterior injection of 0.5 liters of isotonic sea water in 11 minutes: healing without kidney problems. He was run over 5 years later.[2]

He also checked that white blood cells of different vertebrate species (including humans) can only live in sea water diluted with spring water. In any other artificial environment they die.[2]

In 2012, at the University of Alicante (Spain), the normal behavior of white blood cells in isotonic sea water was re-verified.

The therapeutic application of its law to terminally ill people (intoxicated), and afterwards to moribund children, was a total success:

> "The rule is that one hour after the first injection, the child who arrived moribund and who vomited absolutely everything, assimilates a dose of water and one hour later the first

---

(*) Centre de Recherche Delalande: oceanplasma.org/documents/delalande-f.html ; www.dsalud.com/index.php?pagina=articulo&c=1816

dose of milk. In the majority of cases, the suppressed digestive faculty is restored and the child easily gains 500 grams in 24 hours.

(…) Less than two hours after the injection of sea water, his physiognomy is much better and replaces the unforgettable aspect of the dying cholera patient." [2]

Therapeutic results of sea water before Doctor Hamer's discoveries

Quinton and his followers had excellent results for some diseases and mixed results for others.

They got excellent results in the following cases:

- Children with enterocolitis, gastroenteritis, etc. in which the only risk lies in their dehydration. The role of sea water was only hydration (although done perfectly).
- Malnutrition in children.(*)
- For injuries, because sea water is the best aid for repairing the body, since sea water is the best environment for cell life.[3]

For example: as a blood substitute (hemorrhages), as a cleaner for extracellular fluid (side effects of drugs, parasites, lack of excretions

---

(*) Since they don't properly understand what the disease is, they focus on the most successful cases. Jarricot cites the main ailments he treats in his marine dispensary for children:
• Malnutrition (using the nutritive component of sea water).
• Intestinal inflammation (sea water resolves dehydration).
• Tuberculosis and eczema (two symptoms of the recovery phase, for which they use the basic properties of sea water); they don't reach 100% success. As he says "there are stubborn forms of eczema" (which are relapses in the stress phase).
As for pneumonia (symptom of the recovery phase), he recognizes failure (since he tries to eliminate healing symptoms).
www.oceanplasma.org/documents/nourrisons.html

- renal failure, intoxication due to constipation) or nourishing cells (malnutrition) and protecting them (burns).[1a]

They obtained mixed results in the rest of the cases

Because they tried to apply sea water to combat symptoms of the healing phase.(*)

In these cases, they came to the same 'division of opinion' as for any other drug or therapy. (**)

Logically they obtained more cures when the patients were in an advanced state of the disease (they were already in the healing phase).

> "Woman after breast cancer surgery *(if it was a ductal breast cancer, she was in the healing phase),* in full recurrence on the lymph nodes of the armpit and neck *(symptoms of the healing phase),* with painful edema in the arm *(the same)*. Thanks to the marine treatment, the volume of the lymph nodes decreased, the edema of the arms disappeared and her condition gradually returned to normal." *(All of these symptoms being of a healing phase, she would have healed anyway).*[2]

But without absolute assurance, since the patient could always relapse in the grave concern he had just overcome (retracing his steps to the phase of tension).

(*) "In pulmonary tuberculosis (...) a negative result, (...) preceded by a surprising recovery period (...) after which the disease resumes its course." [1b]
(**) "For pulmonary tuberculosis, opinions are divided, but, is it not the same for all active drugs?" Jarricot.
www.oceanplasma.org/documents/nourrisons.html "Psoriasis is cured in half of cases."

Why didn't sea water cure tuberculosis?

Thanks to Hamer, we know that the symptoms of tuberculosis appear when the body is recovering from a previous concern (in the case of the lung, it's the fear of dying).

That is, when the patient overcomes his fear of dying, he begins to have the most conspicuous symptoms (sputum of blood). This brings him back to his fear of dying each time more intensely, since the greater the concern, the more important the recovery symptoms are when he overcomes it.

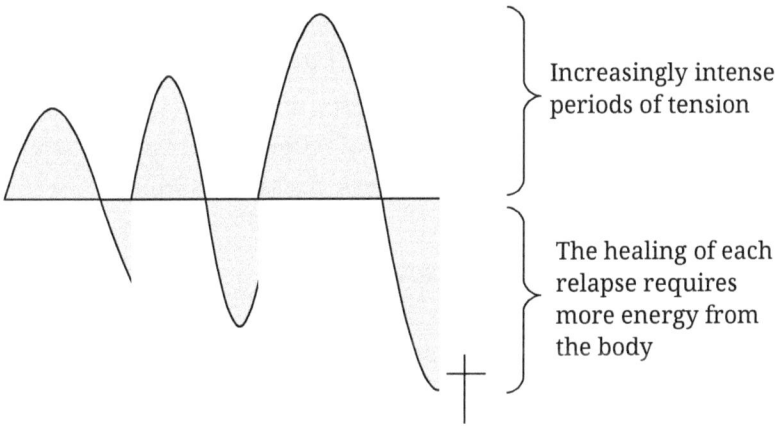

Increasingly intense periods of tension

The healing of each relapse requires more energy from the body

He enters a vicious circle, which ends only when the hemorrhage is greater than that which the organism can support, and dies.

Hamer says that the worst is panic, and sea water can't avoid it on its own. When the patient is already regaining strength (faster with the sea water), panic causes him to relapse into his concern with greater intensity.

Quinton explains it this way:

> "In third-degree **pulmonary tuberculosis**, a negative result, as might be expected, but which was preceded in almost all cases by a surprising period of recovery. The patient, in a state

of complete adinamia and inappetence, with the knee-jerk reflex almost abolished, vomiting all food that he ingests, abundant expectoration, profuse sweats, sternal, spinal, crural hyperesthesias, melalgia, etc., gets up from the first days (second to fourth); the cough, sweats, hyperesthesia, pain subsided at the same time; the expectoration of two spittoons reduced to a quarter, to an eighth on occasions; the appetite, null for months, suddenly reappears and comes to allow up to three or four meals a day, two of them with bread, vegetables, two meats, fruits and desserts. Morphine, previously necessary to ensure sleep, is suppressed after three days; the nights are perfect, when the hospital allows it. After a week, the subject goes down and goes up three floors by himself, remains up for four and six hours. In the most favorable cases, the weight increases; injections are frequently spaced eight days. This period of recovery can last five weeks and more, after which the disease resumes its course." [1b]

Self-purifying power of sea water

When a river is polluted at a point, after a few kilometers, it has cleaned itself up.

(Especially if the pollution it has received is of organic origin.)

This also happens with the sea, but much faster.

This could be verified during the rupture of the main sewer of Miami in 2000, when all its contents poured directly into the beach. After an exhaustive sampling at 52 places on the coast, the official study showed that in a few days the water was as clean as before.[5]

What happens to plastics in the oceans?

Scientists say the amount of plastic waste in the sea has been the same for 22 years, despite plastic waste increasingly being dumped into it. And something made disappear 99% of what we threw. They don't know how, but the waste is no longer in the water.

They think that some fish discovered at great depths might go up at night and eat this waste on the surface. It's the most abundant vertebrate on the planet and with it the total marine biomass is 30 (thirty) times bigger.(*)

Sinking of the Prestige tanker off Galicia (Spain)

Ten years later: "The impact is much lower than expected at the start. There must be very little pollution left. The sea has an incredible capacity for regeneration."(**)

(This is no excuse for continuing to pollute.)

What happens to us when we take sea water as it is, without dilution

Let's imagine that we have 10 liters of fluid between the cells of our body.

We have 90 grams of salt, because the concentration of salt in our body fluids is 9 grams per liter.

What happens when we drink 1 glass of undiluted sea water (100 ml)?

(*) www.pnas.org/content/111/28/10239
www.abc.es/sociedad/20140630/abci-basura-oceanos-201406302004.html
vozpopuli.com/next/45617-donde-esta-el-plastico-que-falta-en-el-oceano
www.fogonazos.es/2013/06/el-pez-que-lo-puede-cambiar-todo.html
(**) www.madrimasd.org/blogs/ciencia_marina/2012/12/10/132925

We will have 10.1 liters of liquid and 93.6 grams of salt (90 that we had plus 3.6 grams contained in the glass of sea water that we drank). (The sea contains 36 grams of salt per liter.)

That is, we now have 9.27 grams of salt per liter, instead of the normal value which is 9.

Normally, our body realizes this excess and urges us to drink.

How much to drink?

Three glasses of salt-free water (or a similar amount of fruit).

That is, 300 ml. Which, added to the 10.1 liters, gives 10.4 liters.

As we have drunk water without salt, or fruit, we don't increase the amount of salt, which continues at 93.6 grams.

But now the proportion of salt in our body is normal: 93.6 divided by 10.4 liters gives 9 grams per liter.

We are no longer thirsty.

Appendix B

How to give subcutaneous injections

There are three ways to give an injection:

- Inside the muscle
- Into a vein (IV)
- Between the skin and muscles (it's called subcutaneous or hypodermic)

These last two can be done:

- With a syringe, if we only want to inject a small quantity.
- By installing a catheter (a special needle with an adapter) connected by a tube to a pocket containing the serum and the liquid medicines that we want to administer. We use this method when we want to inject a large amount of liquid.

For emergency cases, intravenous injection is the most suitable because it produces the quickest effect.

Subcutaneous injections are very easy to perform and have the same effect as the IV, but a bit slower.

René Quinton initially injected intravenously, but went on to do it subcutaneously when he saw that the effect was the same.

This chapter explains how to perform subcutaneous injections, which by its simplicity and its wide applicability, is a technique which we all should know.

(We don't explain the aspects of cleanliness and asepsis because they are of general knowledge and common sense).

Equipment

Syringe and needle (can be purchased at any pharmacy).

The syringe is chosen by its capacity: 5, 10, 20 ml.

We will choose the capacity according to the quantity to be injected. (We may also give several injections without removing the needle.)

Frequently, the syringe is supplied with a needle. These needles are not for subcutaneous injections (they are too long and thick).

It's better to buy subcutaneous needles, which are shorter and thinner, easier to handle (due to their smaller size), and produce fewer skin injuries but have a good application speed, and without the need to press too hard the plunger of the syringe.

Preparation for the injection

Once we have all the equipment, we fill the syringe with the liquid to be injected.

With the syringe upright, aiming with the needle to the sky, we press the plunger to draw air out of the syringe.

If there is a bubble that resists bursting, we give the syringe a few taps.

When the liquid starts to come out the injection is ready.

Where to apply it

It depends on several factors:

- As the area where we prick will be painful for some time, it is best to give the injection in an area of the body that we don't use continuously. It is best to do it on the outside of the legs or arms. Quinton injected into the back under the shoulder blade.
- In the case of animals, let's apply it into the neck to avoid being bitten or gored.
- If the problem is localized (for example: in a knee), it is best to give the injection in this area.

> Let's avoid injecting into an area full of veins, arteries or tendons and areas where there is a risk of reaching the spinal cord or organs.

- To give ourselves an injection, the most convenient place is on one side of the lower abdomen: halfway between the groin, which has a lot of superficial veins and the navel, which has a bigger layer of fat.

> **Application tips**
>
> If sea water is injected undiluted, it will burn for a while (15 minutes).
> So that the burn is not so intense, let's first inject a few milliliters of an isotonic solution and then sea water without dilution.

Using undiluted sea water has several advantages:

- it is three times more effective than diluted
- we don't have to worry about finding trust-worthy water to dilute sea water

Perform the injection

The skin, muscles and bones underneath are not united.

When we talk about the skin, we include all of its layers, even fat. They are all joined together and separated from the muscle below. We can verify it when we flay a chicken.

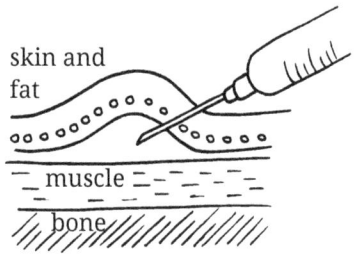

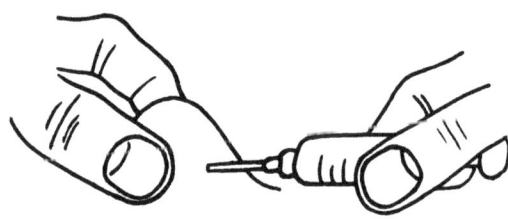

The skin is like a blanket over a mattress (which would be the muscle).

We can move the blanket without moving the mattress.

When we pinch the skin it's like folding the blanket (making a small mountain).

The thickness of the pinch is twice that of the skin (and fat) layer.

The goal is to introduce the syringe fluid between the skin and the muscle (between the blanket and the mattress).

It is very simple.

With one hand we pinch the skin. With the other hand we prick with the needle at the base of the pinch (the base of the small mountain) as seen in the drawing.

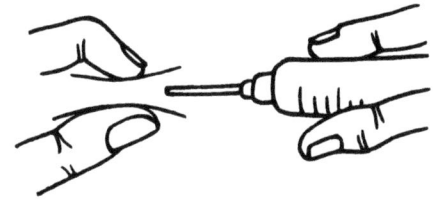

We just have to force a little to pierce the skin with the needle.

Normally the needle is very sharp and it doesn't require much effort. Once the skin is pierced, it is easy to introduce the rest of the needle. (If it is not easy, it is because we are not doing it well. It is better to take it out and start again.)

Once more than half of the needle is inserted, it should be able to move towards both sides effortlessly. (If it's not the case it's because it has not been inserted in the right place, but we can go to the next step which will confirm it.)

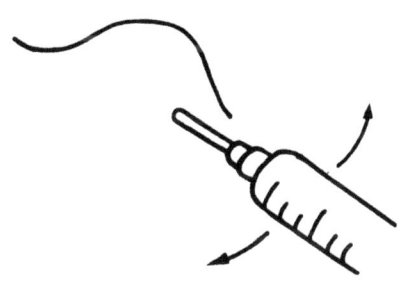

We start to press the plunger of the syringe to introduce the liquid in the place where we pricked.

> If it's difficult, it's because we have not pricked well: either too deep (in the muscle) or not enough (in the skin). We have to take out the needle and start again.
>
> (If we introduce water into the fat of the skin, it remains surrounded by fat and is not absorbed.)

Once we have introduced all the liquid, we pull on the syringe so that the needle comes out.

With these injections no blood appears or just a few drops at the end when the needle is withdrawn.

Depending on the person, it's more or less easy to pinch the skin and detect the separation between the skin and the muscle.

It's possible to inject a large amount of liquid (250 ml) in fifteen minutes without any problem, because the skin expands to make room for the liquid. Obviously, the greater the quantity, the longer it will take for the bump that forms after the injection of liquid to disappear.

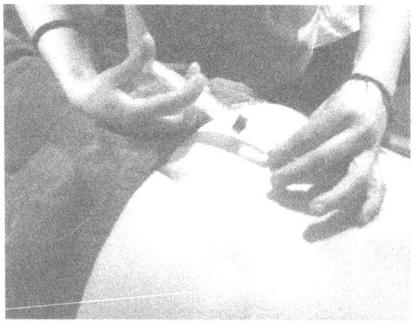

Home treated disc herniation with isotonic sea water injections (see the book's website).

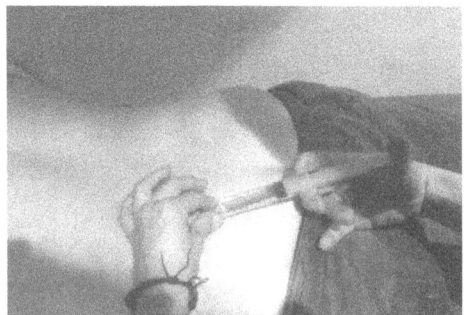

Appendix C

Homemade inventions

« **Ofuro** » (bathtub that keeps the water warm).

Sometimes it's beneficial to take a bath in warm sea water:

- such as for weak or sick people, who could not bear a cold bath,
- or when we are healthy but want to relax.

To do this, we can mount an ofuro at home with sea water.
The ofuro is a bathtub often used by the Japanese.
It is not to wash, but to relax; alone or with more people.
Before getting into it, they wash well to avoid dirtying the water.

It is usually at the maximum temperature that we can withstand without burning: about 111 °F. They use tap water but we can use instead sea water. Like they do, it is advisable that we wash ourselves well before getting into our ofuro, so that it stays clean for a longer time.

> As in saunas, the higher the temperature of the ofuro, the less time should be spent in it, especially people with heart problems or low blood pressure.

We can build a homemade ofuro with a home bathtub or a big barrel. To heat the water and keep it warm, if we have hot water radiators (for heating), we can do the following:

1. Remove a radiator next to the ofuro.
2. Connect the ends of a 10 or 15 m hose to the radiator water intakes.
3. Put the rest of the hose in the ofuro filled with sea water.
4. Regulate the temperature of the water not to exceed 111 °F.

After a few hours of running the hot water through the hose, the water in the ofuro will have heated up.

Although it heats up more slowly, it is better that the heating water doesn't exceed 111 °F, so that the sea water doesn't lose its best properties.

If we insulate the ofuro well, the water will keep its temperature longer.

> The electrical installation of the house must have a differential circuit breaker to protect against any electrical leakage from the heating boiler, or turn off the heating during the bath.

At www.kirainet.com/ofuro/ we can see what the ofuros are like in Japan.

Incubator

In winter, there are people who don't like cold sea water. Whether for drinking, for instillations or for anal insertion.
René Quinton recommended heating it "in a water bath" because in those days there was no electricity.

Now we can build a home incubator that warms up and keeps warm any container with sea water.

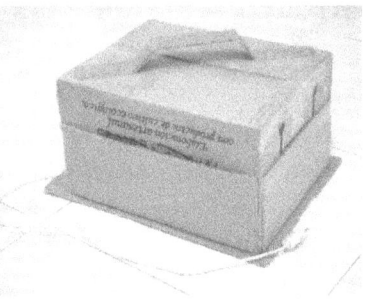

For this we put in a cardboard box a light bulb (non LED) and a room thermostat such as those used for heating systems. We connect them so that the light bulb turns on (and heats), when the temperature drops below what we have marked in the thermostat.

The box must be large enough to contain the bulb, the thermostat and the container that we want to heat.

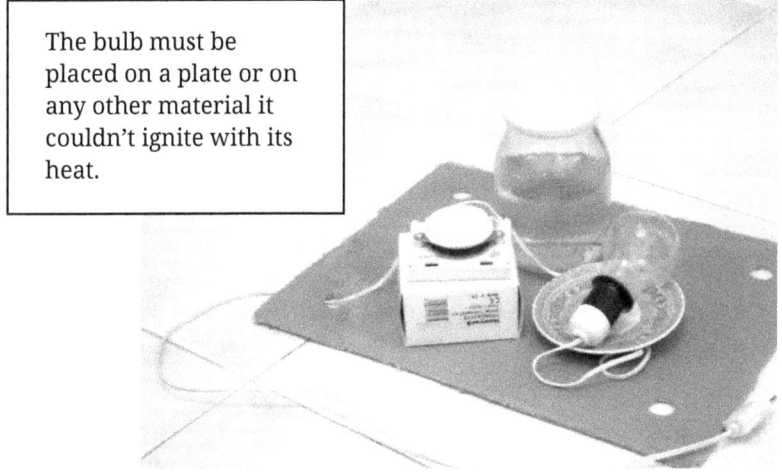

The bulb must be placed on a plate or on any other material it couldn't ignite with its heat.

Instead of heating the water in the "bain-Marie" (which is very cumbersome), we can heat it directly in a pot with the following method: we should stir continuously with the back of the hand touching the bottom of the pot. This way, we know when the bottom of the pot exceeds 111 degrees, which is the maximum temperature that we can tolerate before getting scalded and the temperature above which sea water loses its best properties.

Infrared thermometers

Some thermometers measure the temperature of objects without touching them. They are called "infrared thermometers" or "pyrometers". They measure the amount of heat that anything emits and so they know its temperature.

They use the same principle as non-contact baby thermometers. They don't emit any radiation. They only measure the heat and show their readings on a display.

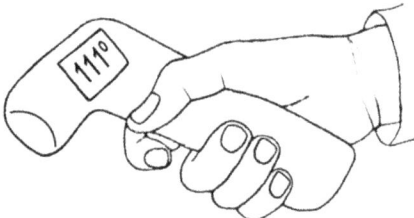

They are found in electronic stores or online (www.pce-instruments.com).

They are not very accurate (they have an error in the measurements up to two degrees), but enough to measure the temperature of food and drinks. They are also useful in the kitchen to avoid overheating food and then having to wait for it to cool down. If we heat it above 111 °F we get scalded when eating.

They are also useful to improve the insulation of our house, to see where the cold enters or the heat leaves.

Bibliography

Books

[1] *Eau de mer, milieu organique*. Livre III: L'eau de mer en thérapeutique. René Quinton. It can be read at the website of the French national library:
gallica.bnf.fr/ark:/12148/bpt6k746094
[1a]: p. 459
[1b]: p. 465-466
[1c]: p. 460

[2] *Le Secret de nos origines*: Les Vertus curatives de l'eau de mer révélées par René Quinton. André Mahé. Courrier du Livre (1993).

[3] *Dictionnaire Vidal*. 1975 Edition. www.oceanplasma.org/documents/vidalf.html

[4] *Dr. Adler*'s book. (in Spanish). The book can be downloaded from the article on teeth in the book's website. There is also an edition published in German.

[5] *El poder curativo del agua de mar*. Nutrición orgánica. Ángel Gracia, Héctor Bustos, Morales y Torres, 2004.
There is also information about the Miami accident in:
drinkingseawater.com/benefits/sea-self-cleaning-power.html

[6] *La cure marine loin du littoral*. L.H. Goizet 1871. At the French national library.

Internet resources

Gallica.bnf.fr
> Website of the French national library. It contains many digitized books from the French pioneers on the medical use of sea water, from 19th century to the beginning of 20th.

P2P networks
> Where we can find a lot of information and some of it not located elesewhere. The most popular are eMule et Kademlia.

www.drinkingseawater.com (book's website)
> With many additional information on this and other subjects (on sugar, salt, etc.)
> The e-mail of the author is:
>
> francisco@martin13.com

Index

Why does the subtitle say "using Dr. Hamer's 5 biological laws on self-healing"? 7
Acknowledgements 9

Chapter 1. History 13
How it all began 13
Why sea water is so effective as a cure 14
René Quinton's research 15
Why did he try with white blood cells? 15
How to make isotonic sea water 15
Summary 18

Chapter 2. Medical and nutritional use of sea water 19
As food 19
As prevention 20
To detoxify 21
To resolve minor illnesses 23
As an aid in healing illnesses 23
For emergencies or terminally ill people 26
How much should we take? 26
Summary 28

Chapter 3. Practical aspects 31
How to take it? 31
    Orally 32
    Rinses and dental washing 34
    By injection 35
    Through the anus 36
    Into the eyes 38
    Sprayed 38
    Washing the inside of the nose 39

Ear irrigation	39
Bath	40
How to get it	40
Conservation	41
Where to buy it	41
Information in internet	44

Chapter 4. Cooking with sea water 45
Drinks and cold dishes. 47
    Citric fruit juices. 47
    Sangria. 47
    Beer. 48
    Gazpacho. 48
    Sandwiches. 49
    Salads. 49
Hot dishes. 49
    Puree of potatoes. 50
    Porridge (oatmeal or cornmeal mush) 50
    Garlic soup. 51
    Fried banana. 51
    Soup 51
Other practicalities in the kitchen 51

Chapter 5. Frequently asked questions 53

Chapter 6. Medical approach of Dr. Hamer 61
How we get sick ?. 66
How is the evolution of the illness ?. 67
    The two phases of the illness 67
    The chronic illnesses. 69
    Relapses before the recovery is completed 70
    Relapses after completing the recovery. 71
CT. 72
Natural relapse at the middle of the healing phase. 73
How to get the original information of Dr. Hamer. 74
Other means of popularization of his discoveries. 74

Chapter 7. Putting Dr. Hamer's discoveries into perspective. 77
The irrefutable evidence. 77
Hamer puts medicine 'upside down'. 78
On the different functions of medical practitioners and therapists. 79
It is necessary to know about Hamer before we need to. 80
Hamer's discoveries are not the panacea (the cure of all the ailments) because it is not a therapy 80

Chapter 8. Breast cancer and heart attack 83
Breast cancer. 83
    Lobular breast cancer. 85
Heart attack 87
    Joseph's case. 88

Chapter 9. Therapeutic guide for the patient 91
First of all: we may decide whether we drink sea water or not 92
Situation number 1: We are well 94
Situation number 2: We are sick 97
Psychological aids to resolve the concern 101
Sea water and cold on the head during healing 102
Other comments 103
For terminally ill people or emergency situations 104
Where can we find help ? 106
Help! I've just had an emotional shock ! 107
    How to resolve daily emotional shocks 107

Chapter 10. How to prevent emotional shocks 109

Chapter 11. Doctor - patient relation 117
Nobody can predict the future 117
Each therapy is ideally suited to a particular malady 117
A treatment or remedy can exhaust patient's energy 118

We are responsible for what happens to us 118
The best therapy is the one that teaches us how to prevent
ourselves falling sick again 119
We can help the body in excess 120
Are we falling into the "halo" effect ? 121

Chapter 12. Medical use of sea water in Nicaragua 123
Summary of the survey 125
Results 125

Chapter 13. A case with initially 'bad results' 129

Chapter 14. Veterinary use of sea water 133
Differences in animal physiology that make sea water administration simple 135
   Case of dog given up for dead 136
   The critical time 137

Appendix A. Scientific basis 141
Extracellular matrix 141
Therapeutic results of sea water before Doctor Hamer's discoveries 143
Why didn't sea water cure tuberculosis? 145
Self-purifying power of sea water 146
What happens to us when we take sea water as it is, without dilution 147

Appendix B. How to give subcutaneous injections 149
Equipment 150
Preparation for the injection 150
Where to apply it 151
Perform the injection 152

Appendix C. Homemade inventions « Ofuro » (bathtub that keeps the water warm) 155

Incubator 156
Infrared thermometers 158

Bibliography 159
Books 159
Internet resources 160

Dedicated to

our blessed mother the virgin Mary,

"stella maris",

"salus infirmorum",

"ianua cæli".

Drinking sea water
Using Dr. Hamer's 5 biological laws on self-healing

1st edition: July 2020
2nd revised edition: February 2023

Original title: Beber agua de mar.
Teniendo en cuenta las leyes del Dr. Hamer sobre la autocuración.

Cover: Enrique Iborra
Back cover picture: Photogram of the video of Dr. Epineuze on Youtube.
Made with free software: Scribus, Gimp, Inkscape and GNU/Linux.

Copyright © 2012 Ediciones Obelisco, S. L. (Spanish edition)
Copyright © 2020 Francisco Martin (English edition)

Author's email: Francisco@Martin13.com

Companion website: www.DrinkingSeaWater.com

ISBN : 9788412442311

This edition is the translation from the 5th revised Spanish edition.

The content of this book is for informational purposes only and is not intended to diagnose, treat, cure, or prevent any condition or disease. You understand that this book is not intended as a substitute for consultation with a licensed practitioner. Please consult with your own physician or healthcare specialist regarding the suggestions and recommendations made in this book. The use of this book implies your acceptance of this disclaimer.

All rights reserved.

www.ingramcontent.com/pod-product-compliance
Ingram Content Group UK Ltd.
Pitfield, Milton Keynes, MK11 3LW, UK
UKHW040833061025
8242UKWH00038B/725